D. Horstkotte and F. Loogen (Eds.)

Update in Heart Valve Replacement

Proceedings of the Second European
Symposium on the St. Jude Medical Heart Valve

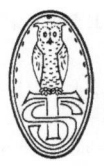
Springer-Verlag Berlin Heidelberg GmbH
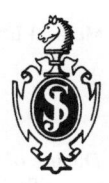

Dr. med. D. Horstkotte
Prof. Dr. med. F. Loogen
Department of Medicine B
University of Düsseldorf
Moorenstraße 5
4000 Düsseldorf
West Germany

CIP-Kurztitelaufnahme der Deutschen Bibliothek

Update in heart valve replacement : proceedings
of the 2. Europ. Symposium on St. Jude Med. Heart
Valve / D. Horstkotte and F. Loogen (ed.).

ISBN 978-3-662-10715-7   ISBN 978-3-662-10713-3 (eBook)
DOI 10.1007/978-3-662-10713-3

NE: Horstkotte, Dieter [Hrsg.]; European Symposium
on the Saint Jude Medical Heart Valve ⟨02, 1984,
Düsseldorf⟩

Copyright © 1986 by Springer-Verlag Berlin Heidelberg
Originally published by Dr. Dietrich Steinkopff Verlag, GmbH & Co. KG, Darmstadt in 1986
Softcover reprint of the hardcover 1st edition 1986

Medical Editorial: Juliane K. Weller – Copy Editing: Cynthia Feast – Production: Heinz J. Schäfer

Contents

Solved and Unsolved Problems in Heart Valve Replacement

C. Walton Lillehei

The proceedings published herein were presented at the International Symposium: "Update in Heart Valve Replacement" as part of the IXth European Congress of Cardiology.

These presentations provide a timely analysis of results with virtually all types of heart valves currently being used.

The observations presented in this monograph by the distinguished faculty point out the considerable progress that has been made in the design, fabrication, and application of prosthetic valves. The opportunity is thus provided to evaluate the performance of each type of prosthetic valve under a variety of circumstances.

It is apparent from these proceedings that there have been noteworthy improvements in clinical results obtained at a number of centers with the mechanical prosthesis in the form of the St. Jude Medical bileaflet, all pyrolytic carbon design. However, results with other types of prosthetic valves, including the tissue types, have remained more or less static. In spite of different modifications of preservation and fixation of the biological material it remains questionable whether important improvements have been achieved concerning durability. Answering this question will take many years.

The five-year experience in the St. Jude Medical multicenter study may be considered excellent. There were no prosthetic malfunctions, and the calculated survival and freedom from thromboembolism probabilities appear to be as good as, if not better than, those obtained with other types of valves, although even longer term evaluation will be needed for final comparisons.

These accomplishments have brought us closer to the "ideal valve replacement" than many might realize. The "ideal valve substitute" parameters of lifetime durability, absence of hemolysis, and near normal hemodynamics have been met by one or more of these modern valve substitutes.

Nonetheless, for the fourth parameter of an "ideal valve substitute" namely, a freedom from thromboembolism, problems have not been eliminated, including the need for long-term anticoagulation.

However, a more careful examination of these remaining problems of thromboembolism associated with valvular substitutes does provide some guidelines for further research that may not be fully appreciated at this time even by specialists active in this field.

It is well recognized by all clinicians that in the life history of valvular heart disease certain pathophysiologic changes occur. What is frequently overlooked is the fact that these changes, particularly atrial fibrillation, chamber dilatation and reduced cardiac output may and do cause thromboembolism from other cardiac sites that actually become significantly more important than the diseased valve(s).

Striking confirmation of this clinical observation has been offered by the recent report of Sage and van Uitert (1). These authors reviewed 140 patients with atrial fibrillation due to *nonvalvular* heart disease who had suffered an embolic stroke. They found that 38% of the

1

patients had died from an initial cerebral infarct. Among 59 survivors who were not anticoagulated, and for whom follow-up data were available, the risk of recurrent stroke was 20% per patient/year for each year of the 9-year study. Patient age and sex were not significant risk factors for recurrent emboli in their data.

The profound significance of this study for clinicians is the demonstration of the very high incidence of thromboemlism in patients with atrial fibrillation and with *normal natural heart valves*.

Thus it becomes very clear that in the patient with valvular heart disease who has progressed to the stage of atrial fibrillation, along with its secondary cardiac effects, even substituting a *normal natural valve* would *not* prevent thromboembolism.

Thus we may conclude that the problem is changing, and that future endeavors to reduce the incidence of thromboembolism in valvular heart patients must lie more with the management of the patient to prevent the onset of atrial fibrillation rather than the often repeated presumption that the "ideal valvular prosthesis" can solve all of these remaining problems.

Reference

1. Sage JI, van Uitert RL (1983) Risk of recurrent stroke in patients with atrial fibrillation and non-valvular heart disease. Stroke 14: 537

Author's address:

C. Walton Lillehei, M. D.
73 Otis Lane
St. Paul, Minnesota 55 104
U.S.A.

The St. Jude Medical Prosthetic Heart Valve: Results from a Five-Year Multicenter Experience

C. Walton Lillehei

During the past quarter-century, hundreds of new and novel designs for prosthetic heart valves have been described. The majority of these have been introduced into clinical usage with great enthusiasm. A few, perhaps ten or less, have withstood the test of time, and in looking back, can be judged as milestones in the development of valve replacement therapy. The great majority of designs that failed were unable to pass the test of time which exposed substantial or even fatal flaws.

Thus, this first intermediate-term multicenter study showing the detailed clinical results in 584 patients who received their St. Jude Medical® (SJM) prosthesis from 4½ to 6½ years earlier under a variety of clinical and environmental conditions, has particular significance in evaluating the early promise of this prosthesis which has been reported upon by many investigators (1–13).

The St. Jude Medical cardiac prosthesis

The design of a rigid bileaflet prosthesis was first described, tested in vitro, in animals, and reported in a series of publications beginning in the mid '60s by Kalke and Lillehei (14–17). The most striking findings from these earlier studies concerned the hemodynamics. They were superior to all other prostheses available at that time.

In 1976 this design was modified and refined for manufacture entirely from pyrolytic carbon (18) which replaced the titanium of the earlier design.

Although there were a plethora of mechanical and tissue valves available at that time, the hemodynamics in most were significantly inferior to those measured for the SJM prosthesis in vitro. Thus, surgeons and cardiologists began to explore the use of this prosthesis particularly in their problem patients such as those with unusually small anuli and advanced myocardial impairment. It was these reasons together with the attractiveness of the all-pyrolytic carbon design that was responsible for the rather rapid clinical acceptance of this new cardiac prosthesis.

On October 3, 1977, at the University of Minnesota Hospitals, this new design was used clinically for the first time in a 67-year-old woman incapacitated by calcific aortic stenosis (19). She had an immediate and dramatic clinical improvement which still persists (New York Heart Association Class I).

Today, 7½ years later, more than 90,000 St. Jude Medical prosthetic valves have been implanted in patients worldwide. The original bileaflet, central opening to 85°, all-pyrolytic carbon valve design has remained unchanged throughout this entire clinical experience (Figure 1).

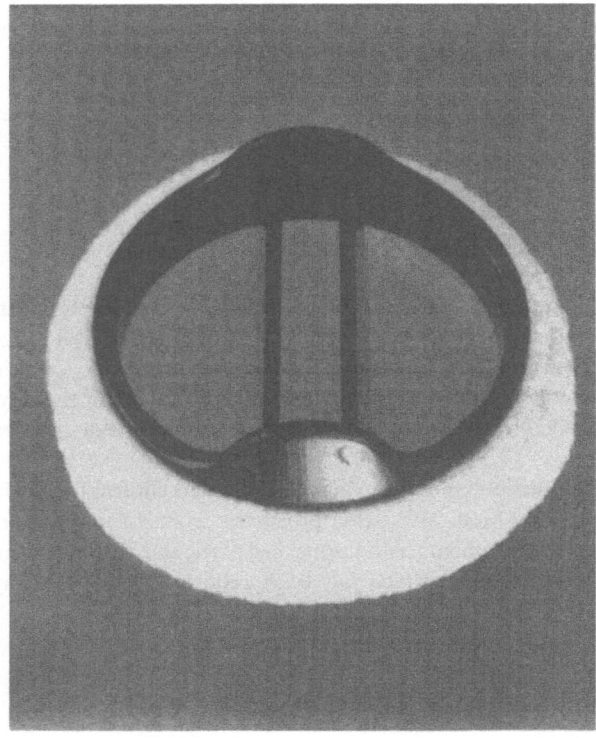

Fig. 1. The St. Jude Medical bileaflet, all-pyrolytic carbon aortic prosthesis is seen from the inflow side in the fully opened (to 85°) mode.

Design of the St. Jude Medical intermediate-term multicenter study

All centers which were early and continuing implanters of the SJM prosthesis with relatively large series of patients and good follow-up procedures were invited to participate in this intermediate-term study of patients operated on for isolated mitral or aortic valve replacement prior to April 30, 1979, (international centers) and prior to December 31, 1979 (U.S.A. hospitals). Agreement to participate was determined entirely by the invited institutions based upon their interest, personnel and facilities. Nearly all eligible centers were able to participate (Table 1). There was no patient selection in this study except for these factors. The principal investigator responsible for the data gathering at each center was determined locally, and was either a cardiac surgeon or cardiologist. Four of the U.S.A. centers listed in Table 1 were also the primary investigative centers for the U.S.A. FDA clinical approval process (approval was granted December 20, 1982).

The surgical techniques were those routine for the particular centers. No special valve orientations were recommended. Permanent warfarin anticoagulation postoperatively was recommended for all patients.

This group of 584 patients comprised 330 isolated aortic valve replacements (AVR) and 254 isolated mitral valve replacements (MVR). The distribution of the SJM valve sizes implanted is portrayed in Figure 2. Double valve implants were excluded from this analysis,

Table 1. Centers participating in the St. Jude Medical Multicenter Intermediate-term Study

International	Principal Investigators
Kantonsspital Basel – Basel, Switzerland	J. Hasse, M.D.
Hôpital Cardiologique – Bordeaux, France	E. M. Baudet, M.D.
Erasme Hospital – Brussels, Belgium	J. LeClerc, M.D.
Medizinische und Chirurgische Universitätsklinik B – Düsseldorf, West Germany	D. Horstkotte, M.D.
Universität Giessen – Giessen, West Germany	F. W. Hehrlein, M.D.
Universität Göttingen – Göttingen, West Germany	E. R. deVivie, M.D.
Universitäts-Krankenhaus Eppendorf – Hamburg, West Germany	P. Kalmar, M.D.
Medizinische Hochschule Hannover – Hannover, West Germany	H. Oelert, M.D.
Universitätskliniken Köln – Köln, West Germany	H. Dalichau, M.D.
Ospedale S. Camillo De Lellis – Rome, Italy	L. D'Alessandro, M.D.

United States	
Hamot Medical Center – Erie, Pennsylvania*	G. D'Angelo, M.D.
St. Luke's Hospital – Fargo, North Dakota*	C. S. Hamilton, Jr., M.D.
Cedars-Sinai Medical Center – Los Angelos, California*	R. Gray, M.D.
Abbott-Northwestern Hospital – Minneapolis, Minnesota	D. Nicoloff, M.D.
Providence Medical Center – Seattle, Washington*	L. Sauvage, M.D.
United Hospital – St. Paul, Minnesota	D. Nicoloff, M.D.
Tucson Medical Center – Tucson, Arizona	C. Maloney, M.D.

* Also primary investigative centers for the U.S.A. FDA clinical approval process

but all patients with major cardiovascular procedures at the time of valve replacement are included. About 33% of these patients had such major additional procedures at the time of their valve replacement. The most common of these was coronary artery bypass grafting (CABG). Other procedures included in this analysis were aneurysm surgery, carotid endarterectomies and various congenital cardiac reparative procedures.

The opening date of this study was October 3, 1977, and the closing dates for the patients' operations have been listed above. The closing date for the patient follow-up for this report was May 31, 1984. All the followed patients in the study were contacted by one or more of the following: office visit, telephone to the patient or family physician, and by questionnaire.

The total patient follow-up was 2,304 patient years broken down to: AVR-1,344 patient years (pt.yrs.) and for MVR-960 pt.yrs. The minimum implant time was 54 months and the maximum was 78 months. The mean follow-up was 49 months and includes all patients who expired or were lost to follow-up prior to the 54th postoperative month.

The probability of patients' survival or freedom from specific complications for five years was calculated by the actuarial life-table method (20), and is given as mean plus the 95% confidence interval. Linearized rates of complications (%/pt.yr.) utilized the methods described by Grunkemeier (20).

In estimating the rate of thromboembolic complications (TE) we have utilized the Stanford criteria (21). That is, TE complications include all new transient or permanent focal neurologic defects (unless they were proven to be due to causes other than the valve), and all non-cerebral arterial emboli. Other pertinent data describing this patient cohort are contained in Table 2.

5

Table 2. St. Jude Medical Multicenter Intermediate-term Study

Total Patient Cohort	584
Lost to Follow-up	25 (4.3%)
Number Followed	559 (95.7%)
AVR	330
MVR	254
Mean age at operation:	54.5 yrs.
Youngest	1 yr.
Oldest	79 yrs.

Total Patient Follow-up: 2304 patient years (pt. yrs.)

	AVR	1344 pt. yrs.
	MVR	960 pt. yrs.
Implant Time:		
	Shortest	4.5 yrs.
		Mean 4.1 yrs.
	Longest	6.5 yrs.

74.5% of all patients were followed 4.5 years or more

Valve durability

There was no structural failure of a prosthesis or its components reported for the entire study period.

Clinical assessment

Improvement in the New York Heart Association (NYHA) Classification provides a subjective measure of a prosthetic valve's hemodynamic performance postoperatively. Objective hemodynamic studies performed upon the SJM prosthesis have been reported from many of these same centers (6,7–8, 11, 22–24, 26) and others (4, 9, 12, 25). These hemodynamic observations, while not a part of this study, have confirmed objectively the consistent and significant clinical improvements seen in the patients' NYHA Classes (Figure 3).

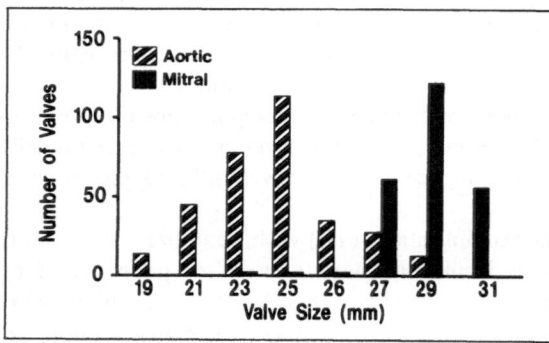

Fig. 2. Valve distribution by size

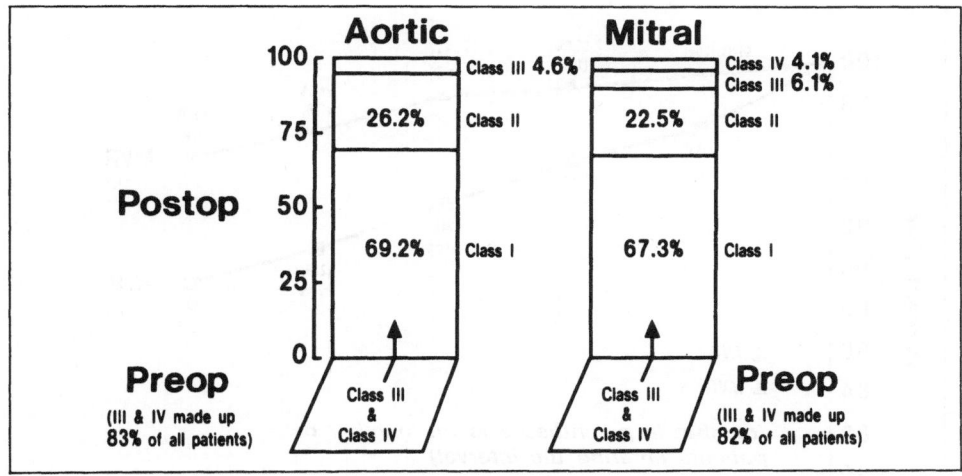

Fig. 3. New York Heart Association Classification

Anticoagulation status and hemorrhagic complications

As part of this intermediate-term follow-up, a survey of the patients' anticoagulation therapy was made, and these results are portrayed in Figure 4. As may be noted, 94.3% of all patients were on either warfarin alone (90.7%) or warfarin in combination with antiplatelet aggregates (3.6%). With the SJM all-pyrolytic carbon prosthesis it was recommended to physicians that the prothrombin reduction could be maintained at 1.5 to 2 times the control level (in seconds) as opposed to earlier goals of 2 to 2.5 times the control (in seconds).

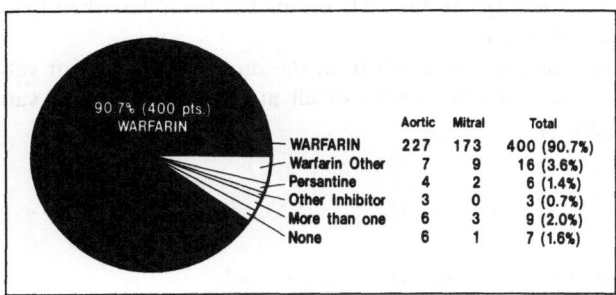

	Aortic	Mitral	Total
WARFARIN	227	173	400 (90.7%)
Warfarin Other	7	9	16 (3.6%)
Persantine	4	2	6 (1.4%)
Other Inhibitor	3	0	3 (0.7%)
More than one	6	3	9 (2.0%)
None	6	1	7 (1.6%)

Fig. 4. Current coagulation status

The number and percentages of patients free of complications due to anticoagulation therapy are shown in Figure 5. In the AVR and MVR patients 89.1% and 95.2%, respectively, had been free of any such complications after 5 years.

The number of fatal complications due to anticoagulation was one patient definitely and two possibly (see below "Patient mortality and patient survival").

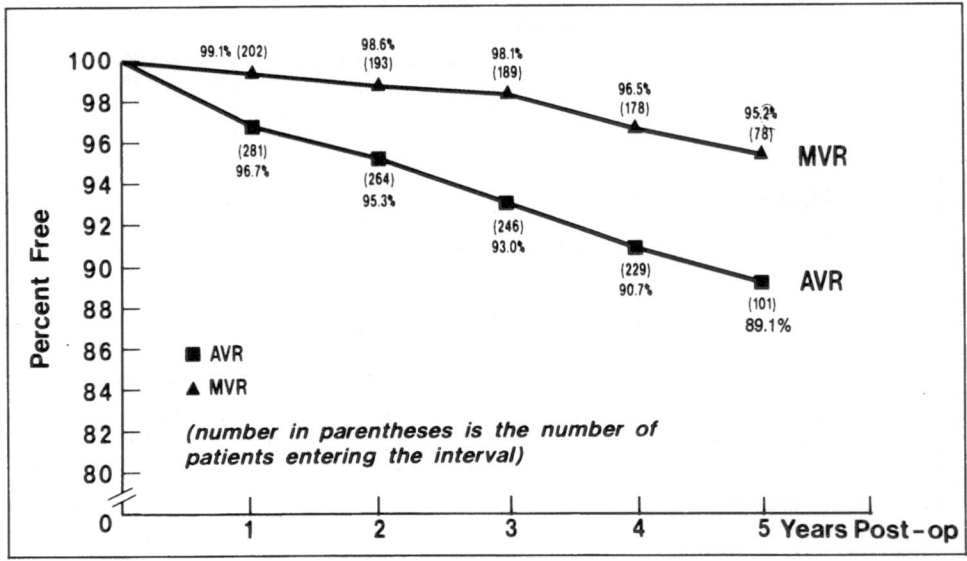

Fig. 5. Patients free of hemorrhagic complications

Thrombogenicity

The percentages of SJM patients who were free of thromboembolic events have been expressed actuarially (Figure 6) and in percent/patient year at 5 years (Table 3). The latter rates were 0.97%/pt.yr. for AVR, and 1.98%/pt.yr. for MVR.

Actuarially the rates at 5 years for SJM patients free of any TE complications were 89.4% for MVR and 95.9% for AVR. The number of fatal TE events has been described below under "Patient mortality and patient survival".

For the MVR patients, there was complete freedom from the dire complication of valve thrombosis during this study period. For AVR, 97% of all patients were free of valve thrombosis up to five years (Figure 7).

Table 3. Overview of results. St. Jude Medical Multicenter, Long-term Study

| Implant Site | Total No. Patients | Mortality | | Linearized T.E. Rate |
		Early (No. Pts.)	Late (No. Pts.)	
Isolated AVR	330	(12) 3.6%	(47) 14.8%	0.97%/pt. yr.
Isolated MVR	254	(24) 9.5%	(33) 14.3%	1.98%/pt. yr.
Totals	584	(36) 6.2%	(80) 13.7%	

8

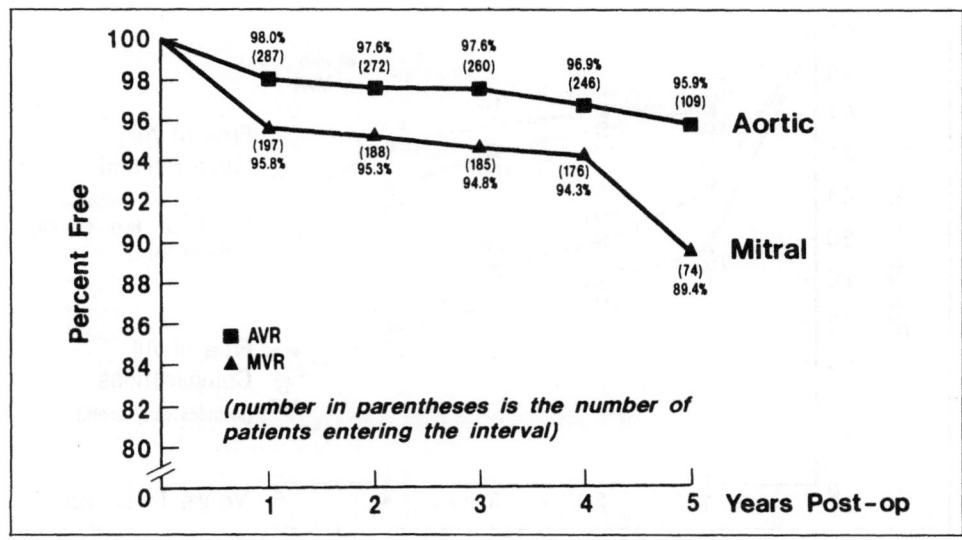

Fig. 6. Patients free of thromboembolism

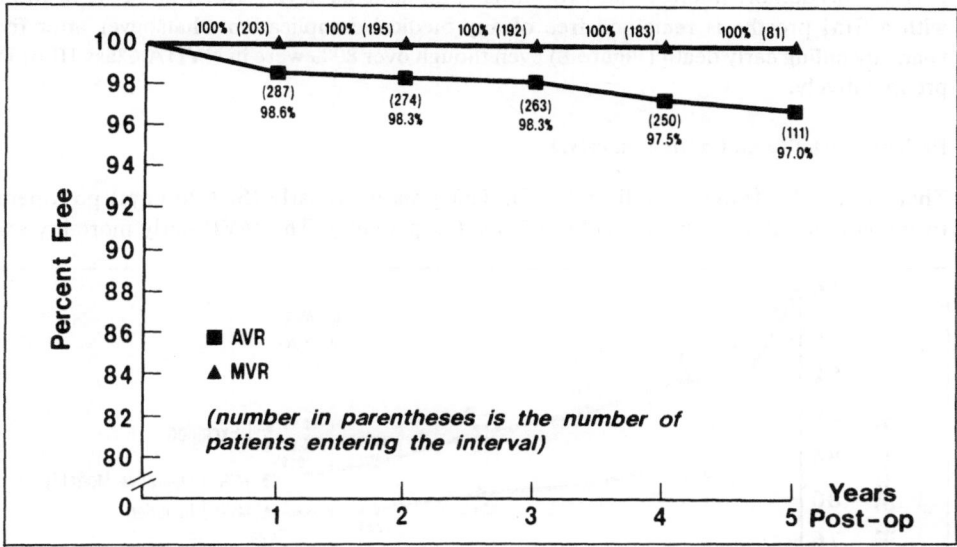

Fig. 7. Patients free of thrombus

Patients free of complications

In this study valve-related complications were considered to be: TE, valve thrombosis, anemia (due to hemolysis), hemorrhagic complications, endocarditis (not pre-existing), and all reoperations or explants. Paravalvular leaks were included when they resulted in reoperations. The actuarial freedom from all complications related to the prostheses at 5 years was 83.0% for MVR and 81.9% for AVR (Figure 8).

9

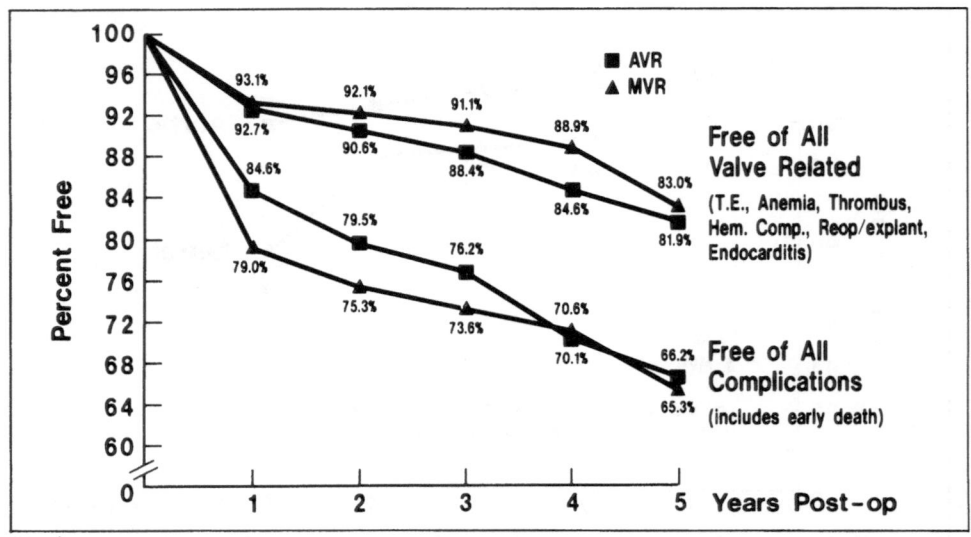

Fig. 8. Percent of patients free of complications

It is of considerable interest that two-thirds of all patients having either an AVR or MVR with a SJM prosthesis remained free of any medical complication whatsoever after five years, including early death (Figure 8) even though over 80% were in NYHA Class III or IV preoperatively.

Patient mortality and patient survival

There were 116 deaths overall (Table 3). Thirty-six were early (first 30 days) postoperatively with an AVR early mortality of 3.6% (12 patients). The MVR early mortality was

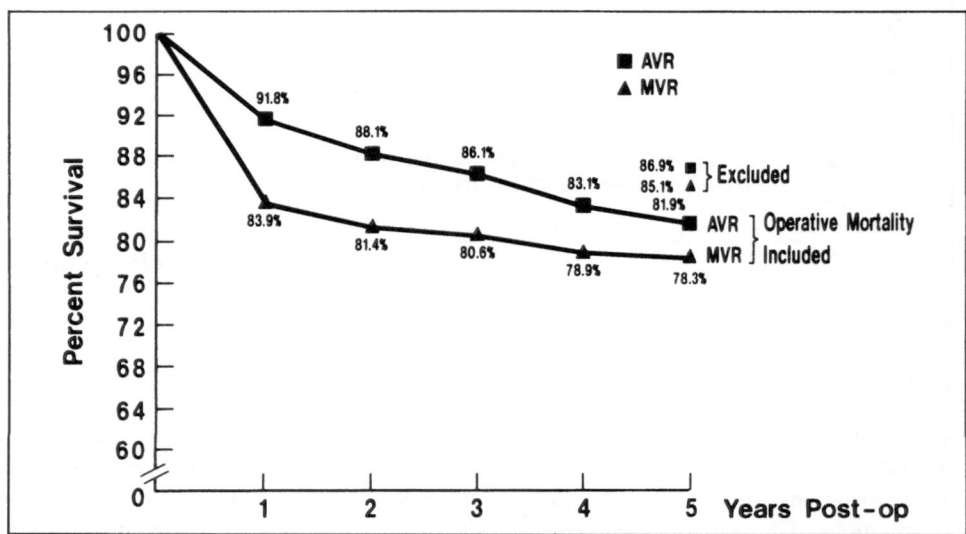

Fig. 9. Overall survival following St. Jude Medical valve replacement

9.5% (24 patients). None of the early deaths in either the AVR or MVR patients was valve-related.

The actuarial probabilities of survival after implantation of the SJM mitral and aortic prostheses, up to 5 years post implantation, are depicted in Figure 9.

The probabilities of 5-year survival for AVR and MVR with the early mortality included are 81.9±4.4% and 78.3±5.4%, respectively. If the early mortality (first 30 days) which is usually not prothesis-related is excluded, the 5-year survival rates are for AVR 85.1% and for MVR 86.9%.

Figure 10 shows cumulative percentages of patient mortality due to cardiac causes that were not valve-related. The valve-related mortality is also shown, and was only 1.0% for MVR and 2.1% for AVR at 5 years.

There were only 9 valve-related deaths during this entire study period, and all were in the late follow-up interval. These deaths were 7 in number after AVR, and 2 after MVR. The two MVR deaths were both cerebral in nature; one was thought to be a TE, and the other was diagnosed as cerebral hemorrhage due to warfarin. Of the 7 AVR deaths, 6 were cerebral in nature, and 1 was due to valve thrombosis in a patient who had stopped taking anticoagulants. Three of the 6 cerebral deaths were believed to be due to thromboembolisms. One of these patients also had stopped anticoagulation. Another cerebral TE death was in a patient with uncontrollable endocarditis.

The two remaining deaths were in patients on warfarin, and appeared to be due to hemorrhage (one had an emergency craniotomy). Whether or not these deaths were definitely attributable to warfarin is not known in the absence of autopsies. Both patients had factors predisposing to hemorrhage (long history of hypertension and advanced age).

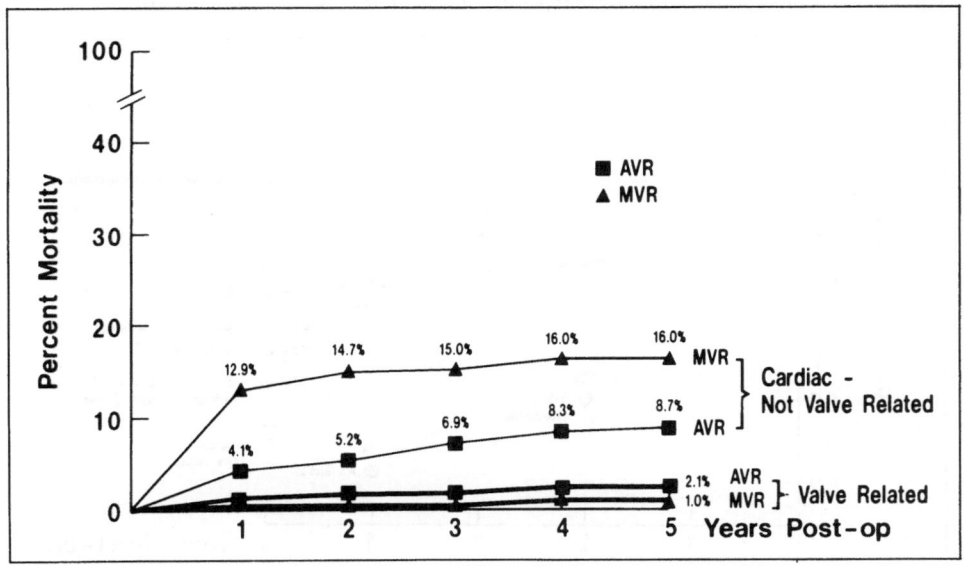

Fig. 10. Causes of patient mortality after St. Jude Medical implantations

St. Jude Medical heart valve – improvement in performance

It is well recognized that complications following prosthetic valve replacement may arise from sources other than the prosthesis itself. However, there is also much evidence from clinical studies over the years which has correlated a better prosthesis with improved survival, fewer complications and a better quality of life (29). Thus, it was of interest and significance to compare the results in this present study with similar long-term studies of the results with other currently used prostheses, both mechanical and biological.

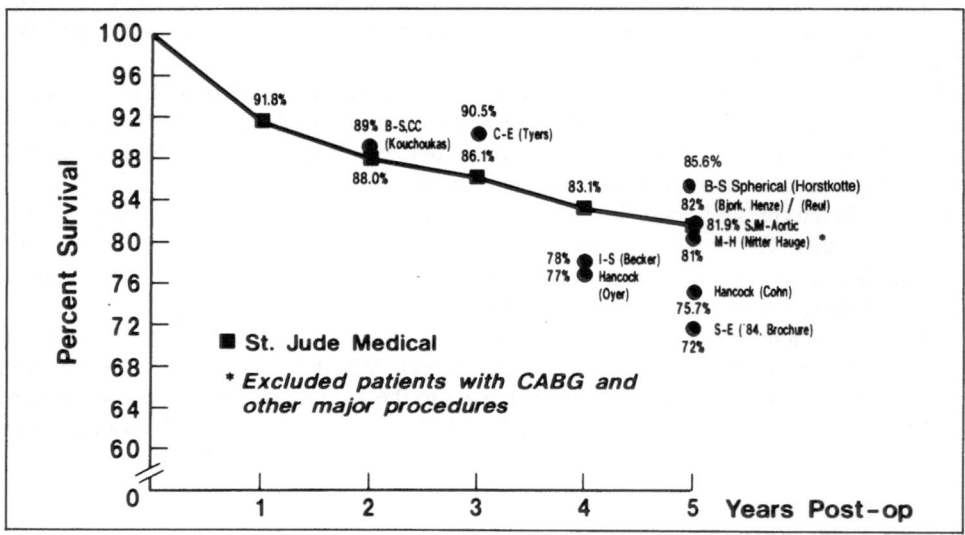

Fig. 11. Survival following aortic valve replacement (St. Jude Medical vs. other valves)

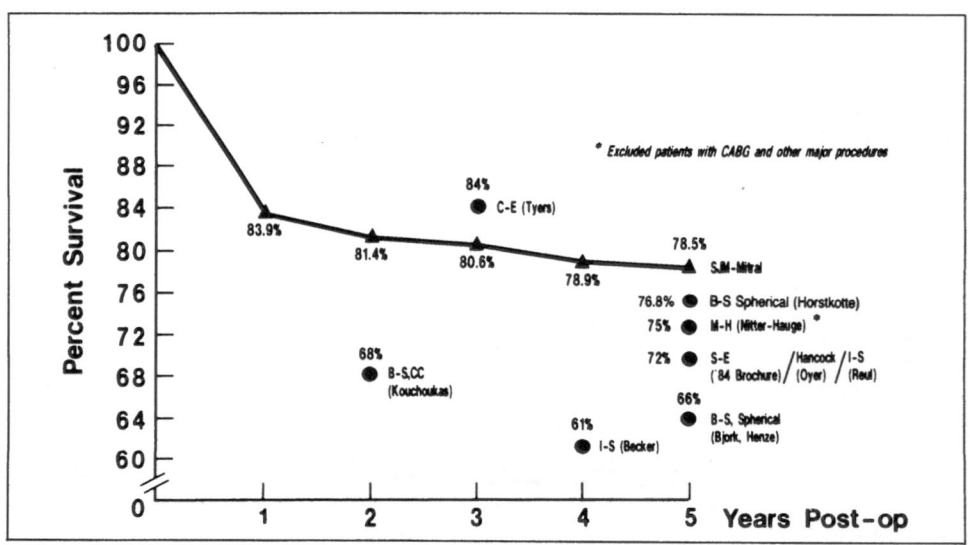

Fig. 12. Survival following mitral valve replacement (St. Jude Medical vs. other valves)

12

The information gathered from these 584 patients who were studied for a minimum of 4.5 years strongly suggests that the unique design features of the SJM prosthesis, including the total use of pyrolytic carbon with its thrombo-resistant properties and great durability, have made distinct and dramatic improvements in prosthesis performance.

Patient survival

Figures 11 and 12 compare actuarially the survival rates of this SJM patient cohort, and those from reports on a number of other commonly used mechanical and tissue prostheses. Table 4 summarizes these comparisons and shows that patient survival after SJM implantation has been excellent.

Table 4. Comparison of 5-year patient survival*

	Aortic Valve Replacement	Mitral Valve Replacement
St. Jude Medical (present study)	81.9% (±4.4%)	78.3% (±5.4%)
Starr-Edwards, 27 ('84 Brochure)	72%	72%
Björk-Shiley Spherical, 28 (Björk & Henze)	82%	66%
Björk-Shiley Spherical, 29 (Horstkotte)	85.6% (±2.5%)	76.8% (±3.2%)
Medtronic-Hall**, 30	81%	75.%
Hancock, 31 (Cohn)	75.7%	79% (6½ yrs.)
Ionescu-Shiley, 32 (Reul)	82%	72%
Carpentier, 33 (Pelletier)	87%	83%
Less than 5 years		
Carpentier, 34 (Janusz)	90.5%	84% (3 yrs.)
Björk-Shiley CC, 35 (Marshall)	89%	68% (2 yrs.)

* includes operative mortality
** patients with concomitant CABG and other major cardiovascular procedures excluded
(±) = 95% confidence interval

Thromboembolism

The sudden occurrence of a TE event in a patient who has been leading a normal or near-normal life postoperatively can be, and frequently is, a devastating and even fatal complication. As mentioned, in a previously diseased heart with continuing rhythm disturbances and without normalization of the diameters of the chambers, not all emboli originate from the prosthesis, but that does not lessen the impact.

Figures 13 and 14 present a comparison of freedom from TE following AVR. Patients in this present SJM study were compared with some of the commonly used mechanical valves (Figure 13) and tissue valves (Figure 14). The SJM mitral valve replacement results in this multicenter study are similarly compared with reports of other studies on mechanical valves (Figure 15) and tissue prostheses (Figure 16).

These data for TE in both actuarial form and in percent per patient year for the various prostheses are summarized in Table 5.

Again, it may be noted that the data for freedom from TE after SJM implantation compare very favourable with other valves. The SJM appears to excel all other mechanical valves in this respect, and the rates are as low or lower than most studies reported for tissue valves. The only significant difference is that 10% to 20% of tissue AVR and approximately 50% of

13

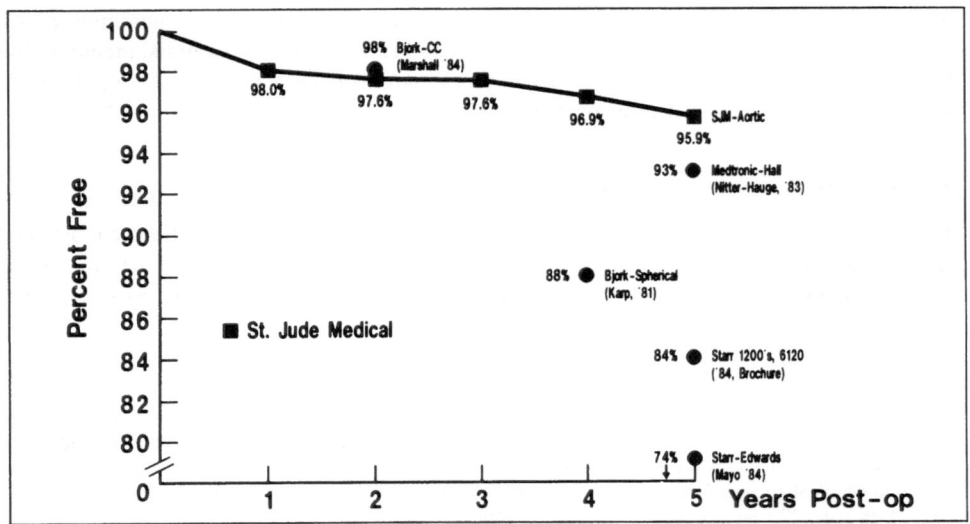

Fig. 13. Patients free of thromboembolism – aortic valve replacement (St. Jude Medical vs. other mechanical valves)

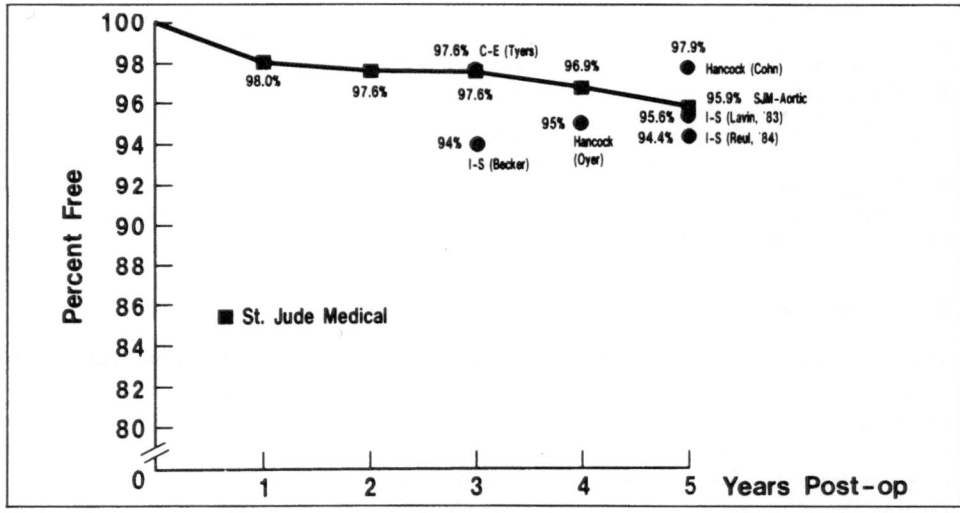

Fig. 14. Patients free of thromboembolism – aortic valve replacement (St. Jude Medical vs. tissue valves)

tissue MVR patients were on warfarin anticoagulants; whereas in this SJM multicenter study, about 94% of patients were on similar anticoagulation (Figure 4).

While the battle between tissue and mechanical valve advocates may not end soon, these comparative figures for thomboembolism clearly demonstrate that the SJM design along with its improvements in materials has been an evolutionary step that has made distinct and dramatic improvements in prosthesis performance with substantial benefits to the recipients. Added to these gains in reduction of thrombogenicity has been the demonstrated durability of the SJM design.

14

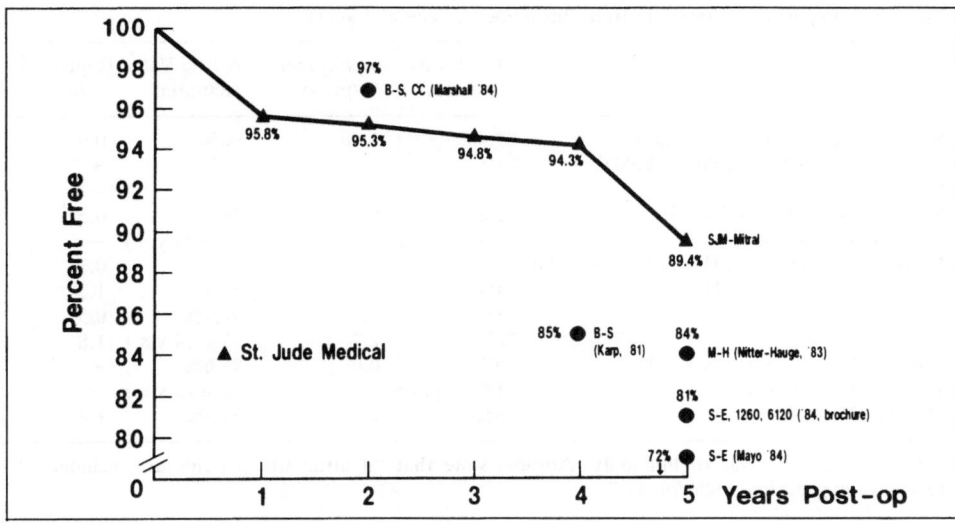

Fig. 15. Patients free of thromboembolism – mitral valve replacement (St. Jude Medical vs. other mechanical valves)

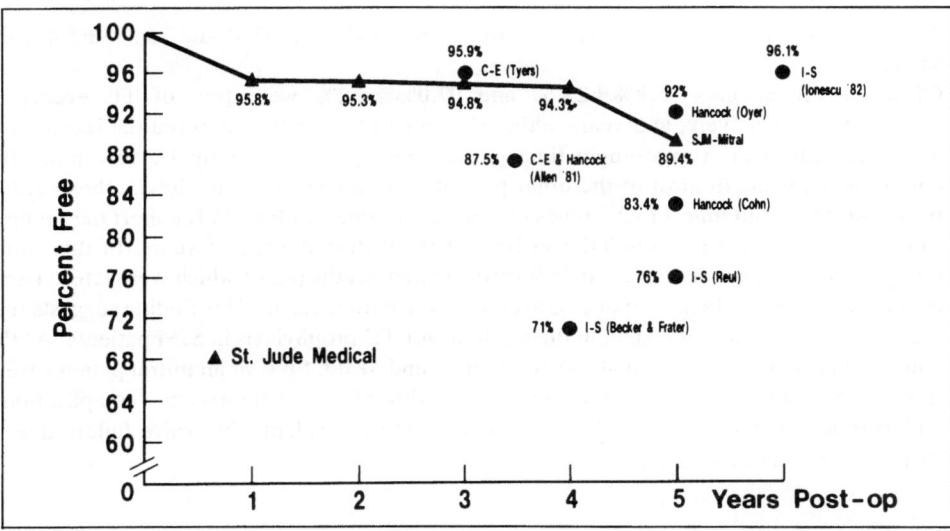

Fig. 16. Patients free of thromboembolism – mitral valve replacement (St. Jude Medical vs. tissue valves)

Conclusions

A five-year (4.5 to 6.5 years) follow-up examination of 584 patients from 17 hospital centers receiving SJM aortic or mitral prostheses has been carried out. This is the largest longer-term clinical study on the SJM prosthesis to date, and the overall results are very gratifying for survival rates, increased freedom from thromboembolism or valve thrombosis, increased freedom from all other valve-related complications and unimpaired durability.

15

Table 5. Comparison of freedom from thromboembolism at 5 years

	Mitral Valve Replacement Actuarial	%/pt. yr.	Aortic Valve Replacement Actuarial	%/pt. yr.
St. Jude Medical (present study)	89.4%	1.98	96%	0.97
Starr-Edwards ('84 Brochure, 1200's, 6120 27)	81%	–	84%	–
Starr-Edwards (Mayo, '84 36)	72%	6.4	74%	6.5
Bjork-Shiley (Karp, 38)	85% (4 yrs.)	–	88% (4 yrs.)	–
Bjork-Shiley, Spherical (Bjork & Henze, 28)	–	4.2	–	0.7*
Medtronic Hall (Nitter-Hauge, 30)	84%	2.5	93%	1.2
Hancock (Cohn, 31)	83%	3.9	97,9%	0.5
Hancock (Oyer, 39)	92%	2.7	95% (4 yrs.)	1.8
Ionescu (Lavin, 40, Ionescu, 41)	96%	0.6	95.6%	–
Ionescu (Becker, 42)	71% (4 yrs.)	–	94% (3 yrs.)	–
Ionescu (Reul, 32)	76%	2.7	94.4%	1.4

* For patients in sinus rhythm only. Authors state that "if atrial fib. patients are included, T.E. incidence approached 4.2%/pt. yr."

The actuarial survival rates at 5 years were 81.9% ±4.4% for AVR and 78.3% ±5.4% for MVR.

Of the AVR patients 95.9% ±2.4% and 97.0% ±2.2% were free of TE events or thrombosis, respectively, at 5 years, although some of the centers followed the recommendation to reduce the prothrombin time in their SJM patients to only 1.5 to 2 times the control level, while in most of the other patients with mechanical prostheses, the goal has been a prothrombin time 2 to 2.5 times longer than normal. In the MVR cohort the findings were 89.4% ±5.4% free from TE and 100% free of thrombosis at 5 years. In this entire group of 584 patients there were only 9 valve-related deaths (all of which were late). Three of these appeared to be due to or aggravated by warfarin therapy. This finding suggests that there may be a need to re-examine the methods for TE prophylaxis in SJM patients. At the end of 5 years, 83% ±6.2% of all AVR patients, and 81.0±4.8% of all mitral patients were free of all valve-related complications (TE, thrombosis, hemorrhagic complications, endocarditis, anemia, paravalvular leak, reoperation or explant). No valve failure due to structural defects was reported.

Acknowledgements

The author wishes to express his personal gratitude to the large number of individuals who have made this study both possible and feasible.
Sincere thanks are offered to the Chiefs of the Surgical and Cardiological Services and their staffs for not only their skilled medical performances, but their generosity in making their data readily available, to Christie DeWitt and Sandy Garlough who skilfully planned and executed the data collection, to David B. Thomas, D. Stat., Kenneth G. Thruston and Maria Brittle for their statistical analyses of this data.

References

1. Nicoloff DM, Emery RW (1979) Current status of the St. Jude cardiac valve prosthesis. Contemp Surg 15: 11
2. Hehrlein FW, Gottwik MG, Schlepper M et al (1979) Heart valve replacement with the St. Jude Medical prosthesis: First clinical results. Thoracic Cardiovasc Surg 27: 187
3. Kasagi Y, Kitamura N, Imamura E et al (1979) A hydrodynamic evaluation of ten various types of mechanical and biological heart valves including Hall-Kaster valve and SJM valve (in Japanese). Artif Organs 8: 140
4. Gabbay S, Yellin EL, Frishman WH et al (1980) In vitro hydrodynamic comparison of St. Jude, Björk-Shiley and Hall-Kaster valves. Trans Am Soc Artif Intern Organs 26: 231
5. Dalichau VH (1980): Frühergebnisse nach operativer Behandlung erworbener Herzklappenfehler. Fortschr Med 98 1: 62
6. Nicoloff DM, Emery RW, Arom KV et al (1981) Clinical and hemodynamic results with the St. Jude Medical cardiac valve prosthesis: A three year experience. J. Thorac Cardiovasc Surg 82: 674
7. Horstkotte, D, Haerten, K, Herzer JA et al (1981) Preliminary results in mitral valve replacement with St. Jude Medical prosthesis: Comparison with the Björk-Shiley valve. Circulation 64 (Suppl II): 203
8. Chaux A, Gray RJ, Matloff JM et al (1981) An appreciation of the new St. Jude valvular prosthesis. J Thorac Cardiovasc Surg 81: 202
9. Wortham DC, Tri TB, Bowen TE (1981) Hemodynamic evaluation of the St. Jude Medical valve prosthesis in the small aortic anulus. J Thorac Cardiovasc Surg 81: 615
10. St. John SM, Roudaut R, Odershaw P et al (1981) Echocardiographic assessment of left ventricular filling characteristics after mitral valve replacement with the St. Jude Medical prosthesis. Brit Heart J 45: 365
11. Yoganathan AP, Chaux A, Gray RJ et al (1982) Flow characteristics of the St. Jude prosthetic valve: An in vitro and in vivo study. Artif Organs 6: 288
12. Duncan JM, Cooley DA, Livesay JJ et al (1983) The St. Jude Medical valve: Early clinical results in 253 patients. Tex Heart Institute J 10: 11
13. Pass HI, Sade RM, Crawford FA et al (1984) Cardiac valve prostheses in children without anticoagulation. J Thorac Cardiovasc Surg 87: 832
14. Kalke BR, Mantini EL, Kaster RL et al (1967) Hemodynamic features of a double-leaflet prosthetic heart valve of new design. Trans Am Soc Artif Intern Organs 13: 105
15. Kalke BR, Carlson RG, Lillehei CW (1968) Hingeless double-leaflet prosthetic heart valve for aortic, mitral or tricuspid positions: Experimental study on replacement in the mitral position. Biomed Sci Instrum 4: 190
16. Kalke, BR, Lillehei CW, Kaster RL (1969) Evaluation of a double-leaflet prosthetic heart valve of new design for clinical use. In: Brewer LA (ed) Prosthetic Heart Valves. Charles C Thomas, Springfield, Il, pp 285
17. Kalke BR (1973) Evaluation of a double-leaflet prosthetic heart valve of a new design for clinical use: A thesis submitted to the faculty of the graduate school of the University of Minnesota, Minneapolis, in partial fulfillment of the requirements for the Ph D degree
18. Emery RW, Palmquist WE, Mettler E et al (1978) A new cardiac valve prosthesis: In vitro results. Trans Am Soc Artif Intern Organs 24: 550
19. Emery RW, Anderson RW, Linsay WG et al (1979) Clinical and hemodynamic results with the St. Jude Medical aortic valve prosthesis. Surg Forum 30: 235
20. Lefrak EA and Starr A (1979) Cardiac Valve Prostheses. Appleton-Century-Crofts, New York
21. Miller DC, Oyer PE, Stinson EB et al (1983) Ten to fifteen year re-assessment of the performance characteristics of the Starr-Edwards model 6120 mitral valve prosthesis. J Thorac Cardiovasc Surg 85: 1
22. Horstkotte, D, Haerten K, Seipel L et al (1983) Central hemodynamics at rest and during exercise after mitral valve replacement with different prostheses. Circulation 68 (Suppl II): 161
23. Horstkotte D, Haerten K, Spiller P et al (1983) Hemodynamic properties of different types of aortic valve prostheses. Circulation 68 (Suppl III): 344
24. Gray RJ, Chaux A, Matloff JM et al (1984) Bileaflet, tilting disc and porcine aortic valve substitutes: In vivo hydrodynamic characteristics. JACC 3: 321

25. Bruss K-H, Reul H, Van Gilse J et al (1983) Pressure drop and velocity fields at four mechanical heart valve prostheses: Björk-Shiley standard, Björk-Shiley concave-convex, Hall-Kaster, and St. Jude Medical. Life Support Systems 1: 3
26. Yoganathan AP, Chaux A, Gray RJ et al (1984) Bileaflet, tilting disc and porcine aortic valve substitutes: In vitro hydrodynamic characteristics. JACC 3: 313
27. Starr-Edwards clinical report (January 1984). Brochure from American Edwards Laboratories, 17221 Red Hill Avenue, Santa Ana, California 92711
28. Björk VO, Henze A (1979) Ten years experience with the Björk-Shiley tilting disc valve. J Thorac Cardiovasc Surg 78: 331
29. Horstkotte, D, Loogen F, Kleikamp G et al (1983) The influence of heart valve replacement on the natural history of isolated mitral, aortic and multivalvular disease. Clinical results in 783 patients up to 8 years after implantation of Björk-Shiley tlting disc prostheses Z Kardiol 72: 494
30. Nitter-Hauge S, Semb B, Abdelnoor M et al (1983) A 5 year experience with the Medtronic-Hall disc valve prosthesis. Circulation 68 (Suppl II): 169
31. Cohn LH, Koster JK, Mee RBB, et al (1979) Long-term follow-up of the Hancock bioprosthetic heart valve: A 6 year review. Circulation 60 (Suppl I): 87
32. Reul GJ Jr, Cooley DA, Duncan JM et al (1984) Valve failure with the Ionescu-Shiley bovine pericardial bioprosthesis: Analysis of 2,680 patients. Presented at the 32nd Annual Meeting of the North American Chapter of the International Society for Cardiovascular Surgery, June 8–9, Atlanta, Georgia
33. Pelletier C, Chaitman BR, Baillot R et al (1982) Clinical and hemodynamic results with the Carpentier-Edwards porcine bioprosthesis. Ann Thorac Surg 34: 612
34. Janusz MT, Jamieson WRE, Allen P et al (1984) Experience with the Carpentier-Edwards porcine valve prosthesis in 700 patients. Ann Thorac Surg 37: 398
35. Marshall WG Jr, Kouchoukos NT, Pollock SB et al (1984) Early results of valve replacement with the Björk-Shiley convexo-concave prosthesis. Ann Thorac Surg 37: 398
36. McGoon D, Fuster V, Pumphrey C et al (1984) Aortic and mitral valve incompetence: Long-term follow-up (10 to 19 years) of patients treated with the Starr-Edwards prosthesis. J Am Coll Cardiol 3: 930
37. Horstkotte D, Haerten K, Herzer JA et al (1983) Five-years results after randomized mitral valve replacement with Björk-Shiley, Lillehei-Kaster, and Starr-Edwards prostheses. Thorac Cardiovasc Surg 31: 206
38. Karp RB, Cyrus RJ, Blackstone EH et al (1981) The Björk-Shiley valve: Intermediate-term follow-up. J Thorac Cardiovasc Surg 81: 602
39. Oyer PE, Miller DC, Stinson EB, et al (1980) Clinical durability of the Hancock porcine bioprosthetic valve. J Thorac Cardiovasc Surg 80: 824
40. Gonzalez-Lavin L, Chi S, Blair TC et al (1983) Five-year experience with the Ionescu-Shiley bovine pericardial valve in the aortic position. Ann Thor Surg 36: 270
41. Ionescu MI, Smith DR, Hasan SS et al (1982) Clinical durability of the pericardial xenograft valve: Ten years' experience with mitral replacement. Ann Thor Surg 34: 265
42. Becker RM, Sandor L, Tindel M et al (1981) Medium-term follow-up of the Ionescu-Shiley heterograft valve. Ann Thor Surg 32: 120

Author's address:
C. Walton Lillehei, M.D.
73 Otis Lane
St. Paul, Minnesota 55104
U.S.A.

Choosing Between Mechanical and Tissue Valves for the Treatment of Valvular Heart Disease

D. Horstkotte and F. Rovelli

Efforts to obtain better substitutes for destroyed human heart valves, starting from the first mitral prosthesis usable for implantation in humans at the beginning of the '60s (1), have led to the development of numerous models of a variety of materials. Whereas during the early years durability was one of the most important requirements for usable artificial valves, the main aims of subsequent efforts were almost physiological hemodynamic characteristics (2) and the reduction of valve-related or valve-induced complications (3). It was soon demonstrated that the probability of complications is also determined by flow-dynamic properties of the prosthesis, which naturally are of paramount importance for the normalization of the preoperatively disturbed central hemodynamics and the postoperative functional capacity of the patients (4, 5).

The two main directions of development – to the mechanical and tissue valves, the latter group subdivided into allo- and xenografts – which brought continuous improvement in design, show that so far, no prosthesis meets all the requirements of an ideal heart valve substitute. On the other hand, mechanical or biological valves, in general, have no superiority over each other. Apart from some rare set backs in single models or production series (6), the mechanical valves used today, during follow-up, fulfil the requirements concerning durability sufficiently. Although tests in pulse duplicators show a limited durability for all mechanical valves except the St. Jude cardiac prosthesis (7), in vivo, this durability fortunately is far exceeded. The hemodynamic properties of current mechanical prostheses are superior to biological valves because of the favorable relationship between total prosthetic valve area and effective prosthetic valve orifice area (4).

When compared to tissue valves, the most important disadvantage of mechanical valves is thrombogenicity, which has been reduced recently by improved construction principles, but is still significantly higher than that of xenografts. Despite anticoagulation and consequent bleeding complications (8), the success of a mechanical heart valve substitute negatively influenced by thromboembolic events (9). The valve murmur, often experienced as inconvenient to patients, is an additional disadvantage of some mechanical valves.

According to the Munich terminology (10) biological valves are classified as xenografts manufactured of bovine pericardium (11) or porcine aortic valves (12, 13) and allografts. Allografts, sometimes designated as homografts, are made from human corpse aortic valves (14, 15), and less frequently of dura mater (16).

In addition to the unfavorable hemodynamic properties in comparison to current mechanical prostheses (4, 17, 18), especially in the smaller sizes (5, 19), the main disadvantage of tissue valves is limited durability due to calcification. Tissue damage is the consequence of destruction of the collagen fiber network, wear of superficial collagen layer, and high shearing forces occurring from obstruction of the valve orifice area. There is a difference between primary valve failures (spontaneous degeneration of valve tissue) and secondary valve failures (from infection). Calcification of biological heart valves results in degeneration and dysfunction. Calcification is at least partially due to the fixation technique and starts in the connective tissue of the valves, from organized superficial thrombi or abacterial vegetations (20). Calcium salt incorporations are often localized at the commissures, i.e. at the free edges of the leaflets (21, 22).

During fixation proteoglycanes and glycoproteins are released from the valve tissue, so that free phosphate bindings form a covalent binding with the amorphic crystalline calcium phosphate. Additionally, fixation releases some parts from the connective frame tissue. After implantation the free spaces in the tissue are filled with plasma proteins which have a high binding affinity to calcium (23).

The expected calcification of biological material is important for the indications for implantation of xenografts, because its extent is influenced by a variety of factors. Parathormone and calcitonine influence hormonal as well as metabolic factors, e.g. vitamin D, and usually faster calcification of biological valves is seen in children (21, 24), where increased calcium metabolism favors deposition of calcium phosphate. Also, early dysfunctions of biological valves due to calcification are documented for metabolic or hormonal disorders like terminal kidney failure (25) and hyperparathyroidism.

Durability may differ distinctly with calcium metabolism and patient age (21, 24, 26) as well as manufacturing techniques and construction principles of xenografts (20, 27, 28, 29). The probable durability of an implanted valve is, therefore, very hard to predict because of the different long-term results after biological heart valve replacement. Additionally, a sufficiently long follow-up period has been documented for xenografts of the first and second generation which are inferior in design, fixation or hemodynamic properties to valves used today (20, 30, 31). Finally, extrapolation of incidences of dysfunctions so far observed seems to be problematic, since reoperations due to valve dysfunctions 12 to 15 years after implantation obviously show an exponential increase.

Because of these influencing parameters, the evaluation of 52 publications on degeneration and dysfunction of porcine and bovine xenografts illustrate marked differences of the reoperation rates reported. After aortic valve replacement the frequency of reoperation due to prosthetic valve dysfunction of about 20% after 10 and 38% after 15 years has been reported; for mitral valve replacements 25% has been reported after 10 and 45% after 15 years. Reoperation, however, does not take into account the number of patients dying from valve failure. The higher incidence after mitral valve replacement can be explained by the higher pressure load of the mitral valve tissue compared to the aortic position (22, 32).

Therefore, after implantation of a tissue valve in patients under 60 years of age, a second intervention is necessary, as a rule. In children and adolescents, especially below 15 years of age, a much higher incidence (up to 10% per patient-year) of valve dysfunctions, compared to adults, has been reported (26, 33).

The risk of reoperation and the psychological problems imposed on the patients, however, are not the only disadvantages to be taken into account when implanting xenografts: the valve function of the prosthesis deteriorates before a second operation is necessary. Echocardiographic studies frequently show a progressive thickening and rigidity of the cusps concomitant with a decrease of the valve orifice area (34) even a few years after implantation. Therefore, for some patients, hemodynamical deterioration and decrease of functional capacity must once more be expected a short time after biological valve replacement.

Besides this slow, progressive prosthetic valve degeneration, valve incompetences suddenly occur by perforation or leaflet tearing, which immediately cause ventricular dilatation due to acute volume overload (there is no compensatory hypertrophy as with chronically progressive volume loads). Without immediate operation the prognosis of these patients is very poor, because of pump failure.

Concerning thrombogenicity, xenografts are superior even to modern mechanical valve models and, therefore, in the absence of other indications anticoagulant treatment for more than 3 months after aortic valve replacement is dispensable (35). For the majority of patients with mitral valve lesions, however, anticoagulation is necessary because of coexisting atrial fibrillation.

The incidence of infective endocarditis of tissue valves is estimated to be higher than after mechanical valve replacement (36, 37). The clinical cause, however, is reported to be less severe by some clinicians (38, 39). Other working groups report no differences in incidences (39). There are various publications which document that infections are most frequently related to the cusps of the biological valve (36, 40), and much less frequently to the sewing ring. It is also documented that extensive destructions occur directly or by secondary calcium incorporations (22, 36). For mechanical prostheses, however, the infection almost always has its starting point at the sewing ring.

Allografts, especially after aortic valve replacement, show satisfying long-term results and good hemodynamic properties, whereas the results of mitral valve replacements with allografts are less favorable (41). The rate of early degeneration of aortic valves amounts to 13% within the first two postoperative years (30) for patients who have a diastolic murmur immediately postoperative. For patients without immediate postoperative incompetence murmur, the rate is below that for xenografts. Later dysfunctions are most frequently caused by tear perforations (30) or ruptures and are less frequent for fresh antibiotic-treated allografts than for sterilized and preserved allografts (42). Calcifications of the valves in fresh antibiotic-treated allografts seem to be less frequent than in heterografts (43). On the other hand, calcification of the aortic wall of allo- and autografts is seen quite often (30, 44).

The rate of valve-induced complications for allografts concerning thromboembolic events is low and their production costs are significantly lower than those of the other valve models, in spite of the fact that some have a short shelf life. The availability of all required sizes, however, is limited at most centers. Altogether, the results of alloplastic heart valve replacements are satisfying for the aortic position, but less satisfying for mitral valve replacement (41).

These advantages and disadvantages of the different types of replacement valves implicate a selection according to age, sex, concomitant diseases, thromboembolic and hemorrhagic risks, social and personal life conditions. However, currently there is no concensus regarding differential therapy. In the following publications, the authors demonstrate advantages and disadvantages of allografts, as well as mechanical prostheses, from their individual perspectives, and these sources may be a help for the differentiated use of heart valve substitutes today.

References

1. Starr A, Edwards ML (1961) Mitral replacement: clinical experience with a ball-valve prosthesis. Ann Surg 154: 726
2. Roberts WC (1976) Choosing a substitute cardiac valve: type, size, surgeon. Ann J Cardiol 38: 633
3. Lefrak EA, Starr A (1976) Cardiac valve prostheses. Historical aspects of cardiac valve replacement. Appleton-Century-Crofts, New York, p 3

4. Horstkotte D, Haerten K, Schulte HD et al (1983) Hemodynamic findings at rest and during exercise after implantation of different mitral valve prostheses with equal tissue annulus diameters. Z Kardiol 72: 385
5. Horstkotte D, Haerten K, Körfer R et al (1983) Hemodynamic findings ar rest and during exercise after implantation of different aortic valve prostheses. Z Kardiol 72: 429
6. Vareia R, Rudensky M (1984) Devices and diagnostics letter 11: 24
7. Clark RE, Swanson WM, Kordos JL et al (1978) Durability of prosthetic heart valves. Ann Thorac Surg 26: 323
8. Horstkotte D, Körfer R (1983) The influence of prosthetic valve replacement on the natural history of severe acquired heart valve lesions: a comparison of complications and hemodynamic findings after implantation of Björk-Shiley, St. Jude Medical, and other heart valve prostheses. In: DeBakey ME (ed) Advances in cardiac valves. Yorke Medical Books, New York, p 47
9. Horstkotte D, Körfer R, Seipel L et al (1983) Late complications in patients with Björk-Shiley and St. Jude Medical heart valve replacement. Circulation 68 (Suppl II): 175
10. Sebening F, Klövekorn WP, Meisner H et al (1979) Bioprosthetic cardiac valves. Terminology of tissue valves. Deutsches Herzzentrum München, Munich, p 405
11. Ionescu MI, Tandon AP (1979) The Ionescu-Shiley pericardial xenograft heart valve. In: Ionescu MI (ed) Tissue heart valves. Butterworth, London Boston, p 201
12. Reis RL, Hancock WD, Yarbrough JW et al (1971) The flexible stent. A new concept in the fabrication of tissue heart valve prostheses. J Thorac Cardiovasc Surg 62: 683
13. Deloche A, Perier P, Bourezak H et al (1982) A 14-year experience with valvular bioprostheses: valve survivial and patient survival. In: Cohn LH, Gallucci V (eds) Cardiac bioprostheses. Yorke Medical Books, New York, p 25
14. Ross DN (1962) Homograft replacement of the aortic valve. Lancet 2: 487
15. Barratt-Boyes BG (1964) Homograft aortic valve replacement in aortic incompetence and stenosis. Thorax 19: 131
16. Puig LB, Verginelli, Bellotti G et al (1975) Homologous dura mater cardiac valves. Study of 533 surgical cases. J Thorac Cardiovasc Surg 69: 722
17. Lurie AJ, Miller RR, Maxwell KS et al (1976) Hemodynamic assessment of the glutaraldehyde-preserved porcine heterograft in the aortic and mitral position. Circulation 56 (Suppl II): 104
18. Morris DC, Wickliffe CW, King SB et al (1976) Hemodynamic evaluation of the porcine heterograft aortic valve. Am J Cardiol 37: 157
19. Hatcher CR (1976) Aortic valve replacement: the problem of the small aortic annulus. Ann Thorac Surg 22: 400
20. Ferrans KJ, Boyce SW, Billingham ME et al (1980) Calcific deposits in porcine bioprostheses: picture and pathogenesis. Am J Cardiol 46: 721
21. Cipriano, PR, Billingham ME, Oyer PE et al (1982) Calcification of porcine prosthetic heart valves: a radiographic and light microscopic study. Circulation 66: 1100
22. Schoen FJ, Collins JJ, Cohn LH (1983) Long-term failure rate and morphologic correlations in porcine bioprosthetic heart valves. Am J Cardiol 51: 957
23. Ferrans VJ, Spray TL, Billingham ME et al (1984) Structural changes in glutaraldehyde-treated porcine heterografts used as substitute cardiac valves. Transmission and scanning electron microscopic observation in 12 patients. Am J Cardiol 41: 1159
24. Thandroyen FT, Whitton IN, Pirie D et al (1980) Severe calcification of glutaraldehyde-preserved porcine xenografts in children. Am J Cardiol 45: 690
25. Fishbein MC, Gissen SA, Collins JJ et al (1977) Pathologic findings after cardiac valve replacement with glutaraldehyde-fixed porcine valves. Am J Cardiol 40: 331
26. Hellberg K, Ruschewski W, deVivie ER (1981) Early stenosis and calcification of glutaraldehyde-preserved porcine xenografts in children. Thorac Cardiovasc Surg 29: 369
27. Broom ND, Morra D (1982) Effect of glutaraldehyde fixation and valve constraint conditions on porcine aortic valve leaflet coaptation. Thorax 37: 620
28. Carpentier A, Nashref A, Carpentier S et al (1982) Prevention of tissue valve calcification by chemical techniques. In: Cohn LH, Gallucci V (eds) Cardiac bioprostheses. Yorke Medical Books, New York, p 320
29. Barnhorst GR, Jones M, Ishihara T et al (1982) Failure of porcine and bovine pericardial prosthetic valves: an experimental investigation in young sheep. Circulation 66 (Suppl II): 150
30. Wallace RB (1975) Tissue valves. Am J Cardiol 35: 866

31. Rossiter, SJ, Miller DC, Stinson EB et al (1980) Hemodynamic and clinical comparison of the Hancock modified orifice and standard orifice bioprostheses in the aortic position. J Thorac Cardiovasc Surg 80: 54
32. Broom ND (1978) Fatigue-induced damage in glutaraldehyde-preserved heart valve tissue. J Thorac Cardiovasc Surg 76: 202
33. Curcio CA, Commerford PJ, Rose AG et al (1981) Calcification of glutaraldehyde-preserved porcine xenografts in young patients. J Thorac Cardiovasc Surg 81: 621
34. Alam M, Goldstein S, Lakier JB (1981) Echocardiographic changes in the thickness of porcine valves with time. Chest 79: 663
35. Holper K, Struck E, Laas J (1977) Herzklappenersatz durch biologische Prothesen. Herz 2: 252
36. Bortolotti U, Thiene G, Milano A et al (1981) Pathological study of infective endocarditis on Hancock porcine bioprostheses. J Thorac Cardiovasc Surg 81: 934
37. European Society of Cardiology: New aspects of bacterial endocarditis. Meeting of the working group 'Evaluation of Prosthetic Valves'. Lyon 1983
38. Quenzer RW, Edwards LD, Levin S (1976) A comparative study of 48 host valve and 25 prosthetic valve endocarditis cases. Am Heart J 92: 15
39. Rossiter SJ, Stinson EB, Oyer PE et al (1978) Prosthetic valve endocarditis. Comparison of heterograft tissue valves and mechanical valves. J Thorac Cardiovasc Surg 76: 795
40. Ferrans VJ, Boyce SW, Billingham ME et al (1979) Infection of glutaraldehyde-preserved porcine valve heterografts. Am J Cardiol 43: 1123
41. Graham AF, Schroeder JS, Dally PO et al (1971) Clinical and hemodynamic studies in patients with homograft mitral valve replacement. Circulation 44: 334
42. Barrett-Boyes, B, Roche A, Agnew TM et al (1972) Homograft valves. Med J Austr 2 (Suppl I): 38
43. Ross N, Mortelli V, Wain WH (1979) Allograft and autograft valves used for aortic valve replacement. In: Ionescu MI (ed) Tissue heart valves. Butterworth, London Boston, p 127
44. Imamura ES, Konno S, Arai T et al (1972) Composite graft of heterologous pulmonary valve and prosthetic tube for the reconstruction of right ventricular outflow tract. Clinical application in four patients. J Thorac Cardiovasc Surg 63: 47

Authors' address:

Dr. Dieter Horstkotte
Medizinische Klinik der
Universität Düsseldorf
Moorenstraße 5
4000 Düsseldorf
F.R.G.

Preferred Use of Allografts in the Treatment of Valvular Heart Disease

E. Struck, H. Meisner, S. Hagl, S. Paek
and F. Sebening

In spite of substantial progress made in cardiac valve replacement including the preparation of prostheses, an adequate valve substitute has still not been achieved. The various types of prostheses developed so far are only partially of the quality of a normal, healthy, human heart valve (Table 1). The predominant shortcomings of cardiac valve substitutes are elevated risk of thromboembolism (1), hemodynamic obstruction (2, 3) and susceptibility to infection or mechanical damage which frequently can lead to malfunction of the valvular prosthesis.

Table 1. Characteristics of natural heart valves and heart valve substitutes

The natural heart valve	Heart valve substitutes	
● Mechanical stability	● High risk of thromboembolism	
● Slow degeneration (if valve is normal)	● Unphysiological hemodynamics	
● Optimal hemodynamics	● Degeneration	
● No risk of thromboembolism	● Fatigue of material	Risk of valve dysfunction
● Low risk of infective endocarditis	● Risk of mechanical failures due to surgical trauma of surrounding tissue	
● Noiseless	● High risk of infections	

Long-term results with valvular allografts

Since the inception of cardiac valve surgery, in a search for the optimum, the human heart valve has been nominated as the best valve replacement (Table 2); traditionally it is called a "homograft" – but according to transplantation nomenclature and in the "Munich Terminology" of 1979 (4) it is referred to as an "allograft" or "valvular allograft". Ross and Barratt-Boyes, in the early 1960s, almost at the same time and independent of each other transplanted an orthotopic aortic valve for the first time (5, 6). The difficulties involved in obtaining the valve and the disadvantages (Table 2), in particular the relatively long implantation time, prevented the widespread use of this method for valve substitution.

Table 2. Valvular allografts

Advantages	Disadvantages
● Near normal hemodynamics	● Not always available
● Low risk of thromboembolism	● Limited storage time
● Low risk of infective endocarditis	● Technique of implantation
● Flexible tissue	● Risk of degeneration
● Noiseless	

Table 3. Comparison of different tissue valves 6 years after implantation

	Allograft	Xenograft
Free of degeneration		
Aortic	97%	96%
Mitral	–	96%
Free of endocarditis		
Aortic	98%	96%
Mitral	–	94%
Free of thromboembolism		
Aortic	100%	98%
Mitral	–	94%
Survival rate		
Aortic	93%	90%
Mitral	–	89%

Individual working groups have, however, concerned themselves with the further development of allografts. This has involved advances in the implantation technique, improvement in methods of conservation and an increase in the experience with their clinical use.

The results reported in the literature in using allografts are excellent, especially for aortic valve replacements (Table 3). In order to give a better survey the data are depicted in a simplified manner according to the results of Ross (7), Shumway (8) and Ionescu (9) and their coworkers. In consideration of other biological valves, the allograft cardiac valves are thoroughly comparable. However, in the period exceeding 6 years after the implantation of the valve substitutes an increasing frequency of valve degeneration has been observed in biological prostheses (10, 11); the increasing degeneration rate seems to be more marked in the use of xenograft valves (12).

In the mitral position, the implantation technique is particularly difficult, so that in this case the experience has been less favourable. For use as an extracardial conduit shunted proximal to the pulmonary vascular bed, the aortic valve allografts can be found to show advantages with respect to flexibility, adequate size and a low risk of thromboembolism (see Table 3).

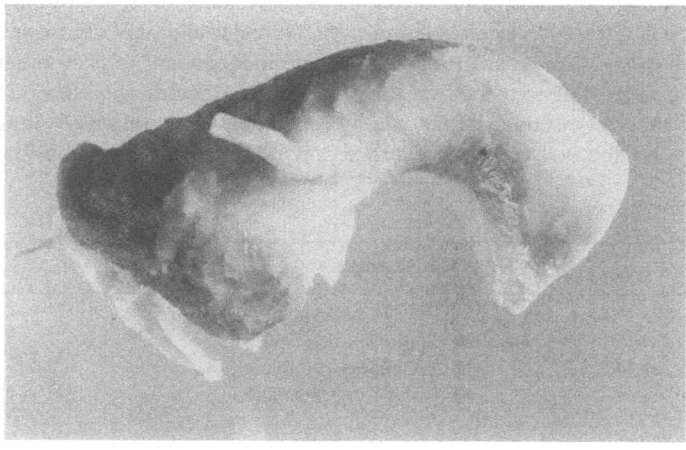

Fig. 1.

Table 4. Collection and preparation of aortic valve allografts, German Heart Center Munich 1982–1984

Total: n = 111	Used for implantation n = 53		Not used for implantation n = 58	
	Range	Mean	Range	Mean
Diameter of the valve (mm)	15–26	20.7	14–26	21.3
Diameter of the aorta (mm)	12–26	17.4	12–23	17.8
Length (mm)	5–70	25.1	10–60	23.8
Age of the donor (years)	7–35	20.6	6–34	21.0
Preparation after death (hours)	0–36	20.9	0–36	20.6
Use after collection (days)	9–31	18.1	–	–

Experience with valvular allografts at the German Heart Center in Munich

In the German Heart Center in Munich we began treating congenital lesions with pathologic pulmonary blood flow by using aortic valve allografts. Currently, our own experience with this method is based on its use for two years.

To obtain the allografts we use the method of Ross (5) (Figure 1): the valve, together with a segment of the aorta of varying length, are obtained and placed in an antibiotic-nutritive solution and stored under bacteriological control for a maximum of four weeks. In our two-year experience, 111 allografts have been obtained and prepared. Fifty-three allografts were implanted in 53 patients. Fifty-eight allografts had to be discarded (Table 4), since no patient of compatible size was available or because a portion of the valve was contaminated or damaged. More recently, in the last half-year, of 17 prepared allografts only 4 have not been used.

The indication for the use of allografts (Table 5) in 2 of the 53 patients was reconstruction of the left ventricular outflow tract; otherwise they were used exclusively for anomalies in the region of the right heart including the main pulmonary artery. These anomalies were a Fallot with pulmonary atresia, ventricular septal defect with pulmonary stenosis, truncus arteriosus, single ventricle and tricuspid atresia.

Table 5. Type of procedure with the use of aortic valve allograft, German Heart Center Munich 1982–1984

	Number
LV–AO conduit	
LV–apex outlet (AS)	1
Aortic root replacement (AI)	1
RV–PA conduit	
Tetralogy of Fallot (+ PS)	10
Pulmonary valve atresia + VSD (+ TGA)	12
Truncus arteriosus	19
RA–RV(PA) conduit	
Tricuspid atresia	6
Single ventricle	4
Total number up to June 1984	53

Table 6. Previous palliative or corrective operations in 32 patients

Type of procedure	Number
Blalock–Taussig shunt	11
Waterston shunt	3
Other central aorto–pulmonary shunts	3
Pulmonary commissurotomy	1
Palliative RV–PA conduit	2
Blalock–Hanlon procedure	2
Aortic valvuloplasty	1
Aortic valve commissurotomy	1
Ligation of patent ductus arteriosus	1
Corrective RV–PA conduit (+VSD closure)	3
Pulmonary artery banding	7
Fallot correction	5
Truncus arteriosus correction	3
RA–RV conduit	1
Explorative thoracotomy	1
Total number up to June 1984	45

In 32 patients palliative interventions had been previously performed (Table 6). In 8 patients the implantation of an aortic valve conduit was only a conduit exchange in the presence of previously performed total correction with a xenograft or an allograft conduit. In addition to the conduit exchange, a ventricular septal defect was closed in two patients. In 2 cases, the conduit was palliative in the presence of ventricular septal defect with pulmonary atresia and a pulmonary vascular bed of inadequate size. The hospital mortality in these patients was 7.5% (Table 7). All operations with a fatal outcome had been performed on an emergency basis. One patient with left ventricular outflow tract reconstruction died in another hospital of unknown causes 10 months postoperatively. One further patient who had undergone surgery for correction of truncus arteriosus died days after he has been discharged due to pulmonary hypertension and myocardial failure. Thus, the total mortality was 11.3%. The mean follow-up period is approximately one year with a range from 1 to 24 months. Six of the patients subsequently underwent additional cardiac surgery for reoperation of previously corrected additional cardiac defects. Of the survivors 93.6% improved after surgery, some markedly. One patient's condition deteriorated progressively because of fixed pulmonary hypertension. Two other patients required reoperation due to residual ventricular septal defects. Regurgitation across the allograft was not observed in any of the cases.

Right bundle branch block after additional ventricular septal defect closure was seen in a group of 43 patients or 28% of all cases (Table 7). Calcification of the aortic wall – but not of the aortic valve – was detected radiologically in 6 cases (11.3%). In 2 cases calcification occurred as early as 3 months postoperatively. Extensive, markedly rigid calcification was found in a replaced allograft, which had been implanted 12 years previously. Other complications specific to allografts have not been observed although in ten cases the allograft required lengthening intraoperatively with a vascular prosthesis.

In conclusion our own experience with aortic valve allografts, similar to that reported in the literature, is promising. In the near future we also plan to begin orthotopic transplantation of such allografts. The valvular allograft may appear superior to xenografts in terms of longevity, however, there is a definite risk of degeneration associated with the use of this

Table 7. Valvular allografts for surgical treatment of congenital malformations, German Heart Center Munich 1982–1984

Patients (number)	53
Age (mean) (years)	7.3
Weight (mean) (kg)	22.3
Hospital mortality (%)	7.5
Overall mortality (%)	11.3
Follow-up (months)	570
Follow–up/patient (months)	11.8
Right bundle block (%)	28.0
Improved condition (%)	93.6
Calcification of allograft (%)	11.3
Allograft dysfunction (%)	0

valve type. In childhood, this disadvantage is made up for by the particular advantages of allografts as compared with mechanical prostheses and xenografts. Improved methods of conservation, obtaining the allografts from hemodynamically stable donors after cerebral death with improved tissue vitality, shortened storage times, consideration of immunologic compatibility, as well as the possibility of immunosuppressive treatment of the recipient, can contribute to the improvement of long-term results after implantation of allografts. The use of allografts, however, is subject to the limitations of their availability.

References

1. Horstkotte D, Körfer R, Seipel L et al (1983) Late complications in patients with Björk-Shiley and St. Jude Medical heart valve replacement. Circulation 68 (Suppl II): 175
2. Horstkotte D, Haerten K, Körfer R et al (1983) Hemodynamic findings at rest and during exercise after implantation of different aortic valve prostheses. Z Kardiol 72:429
3. Horstkotte D, Haerten K, Seipel L et al (1983) Central hemodynamics at rest and during exercise after mitral valve replacement with different prostheses. Circulation 68 (Suppl II):161
4. Sebening F, Klövekorn WP, Meisner H et al (1979) Bioprosthetic cardiac valves. Terminology of tissue valves. Deutsches Herzzentrum München, Munich, p 405
5. Ross DN (1962) Homograft replacement of the aortic valve. Lancet 2, 487
6. Barratt-Boyes BG (1964) Homograft aortic valve replacement in aortic incompetence and stenosis. Thorax 19: 131
7. Ross DN, Martelli V, Wain WH (1979) Allograft and autograft valves used for aortic valve replacement. In: Ionescu MI (ed) Tissue Heart Valves. Butterworths, London, p 127
8. Oyer PE, Miller DC, Stinson EB et al (1980) Clinical durability of the Hancock porcine bioprosthetic valve. J Thorac Cordiovasc Surg 80: 824
9. Ionescu MI, Tandon AP, Mary DAS et al (1977) Heart valve replacement with the Ionescu-Shiley pericardial xenograft. J Thorac Cordiovasc Surg 73:31
10. Oyer PE, Stinson EB (1983) Biological Valves. In: Glenn WL, Baue AE, Geha AS, et al (eds) Thoracic and Cordiovascular Surgery. Appleton-Century-Crofts, Norwalk, p 1362
11. Schoen FJ, Collins JJ, Cohn LH (1983) Long-term failure rate and morphologic correlations in porcine bioprosthetic heart valves. Am J Cardiol 51:957
12. Wallace RB (1975) Tissue valves. Am J Cardiol 35:866

Authors' address:
Professor E. Struck
Deutsches Herzzentrum
Lothstraße 11
8000 München
F.R.G.

The Use of Mechanical Valves in the Treatment of Valvular Heart Disease

L. C. D'Alessandro, C. Narducci, A. Pucci, G. Rabitti, B. Ragusa, P. Mamone and M. Benhar

Some 25 years after the implantation of a substitute cardiac valve, the choice of a prosthesis still remains difficult and controversial. However, progress has been made in creating new models of cardiac valvular prostheses and we are somewhat closer to the "ideal prosthesis" which should have physiological hemodynamics, be thromboresistant, and have lifetime durability (1). After using ball, disc and biological prostheses, we began at the San Camillo Hospital in Rome to use the St. Jude Medical® (SJM) bileaflet valve in 1978, after we had learned from in vitro studies about the favorable hemodynamics of the valve (2). This report will give clinical and practical data on this prosthesis from the Cardiac Surgery Center at San Camillo Hospital in Rome.

Experience with the St. Jude Medical® prosthesis

Our clinical use of the SJM heart valve started in November 1978. At that time, we were favorably impressed by the design and structural characteristics of the valve. The good hemodynamics of the prosthesis are made possible by the two leaflets already opening at a low pressure gradient of less than 1 mm Hg in parallel at angles of 85 degrees (2) providing central near laminar flow with flat velocity profiles, low shear rates and low transprosthetic pressure gradients (3–5). All of the rigid structures (ring and leaflets) are made from pyrolytic carbon and provide increased resistance to fatigue and improved thrombo-resistance. The low profile of the prosthesis does not obstruct the left ventricular outflow tract in the mitral position. In 66 months of use (November 1978 to April 1984), 987 patients received 1,168 SJM prostheses in various positions. Isolated valvular implants were distributed as follows: 328 aortic with an operative mortality (death within 30 days postoperative) of 5%, 473 mitral with 10% operative mortality; 3 tricuspid implants with an operative mortality of 33.3%. These 3 patients were drug addicts with infective endocarditis of their natural tricuspid valves. Double valve implants were as follows: 171 aortic and mitral valves with an operative mortality of 6%, 1 aortic and tricuspid because of infective endocarditis without mortality; 7 mitral and tricuspid with an operative mortality of 14.3%. Three patients had triple valve replacement in the aortic, mitral and tricuspid positions with an operative mortality of 66%. One patient received a mitral prosthesis and a SJM aortic valve conduit.

Selection of valve size and operative techniques

Since 1980 we have used a formula which correlates the orifice diameter of the prosthesis in millimeters (mm) with that of the body surface in square meters (m^2) to obtain efficient hemodynamic results in our patients (see Table 1). The use of this formula has produced valid hemodynamic results, even if a prosthesis one size smaller relative to the body surface

Table 1. Correlation between body surface and prosthetic valve size

Body surface (m²)	SJM aortic valve size (mm)	SJM mitral valve size (mm)
1.00–1.40	19	23
1.41–1.50	21	25
1.51–1.60	23	27
1.61–1.70	25	29
1.71–1.80	27	31
1.81–1.90	29	31
1.91–2.00	31	–

had to be implanted. The transprosthetic systolic gradients in the aortic valves have always been less than 10 mm Hg at rest, even with the small prosthetic sizes.

We have never found it necessary to implant a prosthesis less than 21 mm in diameter in the aortic position. However, we were forced to use the Konno procedure (6) for aortoplasty in two patients to implant a prosthesis of adequate size according to our correlation formula. These patients had previous operations, and were highly symptomatic with a residual transprosthetic aortic gradient greater than 50 mm Hg before reoperation. We also use a correlation formula to determine prosthesis size for the mitral position (see Table 1). Use of this formula has resulted in diastolic gradients in the mitral position always less than 3 mm Hg at rest.

We advise against implanting a biological prosthesis in the mitral position and a SJM valve in the aortic position when double valve replacement is indicated. The leaflets of the SJM valve may be impeded by one of the stents of the bioprosthesis which protrude into the outflow tract of the left ventricle in the subaortic position. We lost a patient who had such a bioprosthesis in the mitral position to avoid anticoagulation and a SJM valve in the aortic position because of a small aortic anulus. To avoid any interference with leaflet motion, we orient one pivot guard at the commissure between the noncoronary cusp and the right coronary cusp. Also, we take particular care to see that calcium fragments do not protrude from the aortic anulus after the removal of the aortic cusps. For this same reason, the use of anchorage sutures with pledgets in the subaortic position is avoided.

We implant the SJM mitral prosthesis in the anatomical position, i.e., with the valve's leaflets parallel to the natural commissure. Particular care must be taken to remove the secondary chordae tendineae from the lateral wall of the left ventricle in the subcommissural positions because they may cause leaflet interference. The implant of a SJM valve larger than that indicated in Table 1 should be avoided in patients with replacement for valve incompetence or combined lesions because the resulting decrease of the left ventricular diameters postoperatively may impede leaflet motion and result in dysfunction.

Out of the 987 SJM valve implants, 174 (17.5%) patients had associated procedures performed: removal of left atrium thrombosis (n=55), tricuspid correction (n=59), aortocoronary bypass (n=27), subaortic stenosis correction (n=9), atrial septal defect closure (n=8), Konno aortoplasty (n=2), and other procedures (n=14).

Clinical improvement and hemodynamic performance

Our follow-up was completed on 534 of the 845 patients who were operated upon up to December 31, 1983, i.e., a follow-up rate slightly less than 70%.
The low rate of follow-up was due to the fact that 20–25% of patients are of foreign nationality and follow-up information was more difficult to obtain. Follow-up was for a minimum of 6 months and a maximum of 66 months, with a mean of 32 months. Factors influencing the postoperative improvement of a patient according to the New York Heart Association's (NYHA) classification (7) are in most cases the seriousness of the patient's valvular disease and the consecutive, continuing involvement of the myocardial function of both ventricles. Two other important factors are the seriousness of the pulmonary vascular disease, i.e., a continuing increase of pulmonary vascular resistance, and the functional involvement of other organs, in particular the lungs, liver and kidneys.
Preoperative evaluation showed 10% of patients followed were in Class II, 70% in Class III and 20% in Class IV. Postoperatively: 100% of patients in Class II moved to Class I; 70% in Class III moved to Class I and 30% moved to Class II; 68% of patients in Class IV moved to Class II, 30% moved to Class III and only 2% remained in Class IV (Figure 1).
After implantation of a valvular prosthesis, the clinical improvement correlates with the hemodynamics of the prosthesis (8). Using the patients' improvement in NYHA Classification as a measure of hemodynamic improvement, 98% improved hemodynamically postoperatively. For the remaining 2%, the irreversability of ventricular damage rather than the valve's performance may be responsible for the lack of improvement.

Valve durability and reoperation rate

Survival and late mortality rates attest to the durability of the SJM valve. No cause of death was due to prosthetic fatigue or dysfunction.
Between January and May 1984 we operated on only one patient, 6 months postoperatively, for thrombosis of the SJM valve. The reasons for the dysfunction as determined at reoperation were residual chordae tendineae, excessive prosthesis size and an antianatomical orientation. During the same period 54 patients with bioprostheses implanted 2 to 6 years previously were reoperated for valve dysfunction. By position these bioprostheses reoperations were: mitral 38, aortic 15 and tricuspid 1. Even if this comparison may not be statistically acceptable, it is significant that we started to implant SJM valves and xenografts at about the same time in 1978 and up to the end of 1983 in about the same frequency.

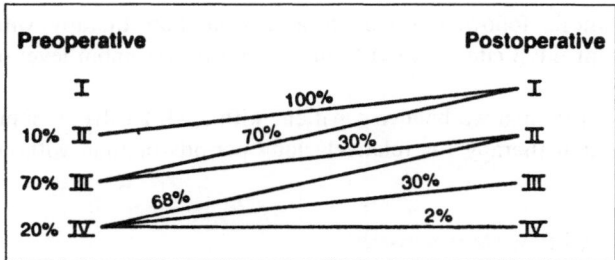

Fig. 1. New York Heart Association Class improvement in 534 patients after St. Jude Medical mitral, aortic or multivalvular implants.

Table 2. Distribution of 6 cases of thromboembolism in 534 patients with SJM valves

Valve position	Location of thromboembolism	Months postimplant	Outcome
Aortic/mitral	Femoral	6	Alive
Aortic	Humeral	8	Alive
Aortic	Femoral	12	Alive
Aortic	Cerebral	12	Alive
Mitral	Cerebral	12	Alive
Mitral	Cerebral	12	Death
Overall thromboembolic rate		0.48%/pat. year	

Expressed statistically in the same five-month period the incidence of valve dysfunction for the SJM to the biological prostheses was 1:54 (total dysfunctions: 55; bioprostheses: 54 or 98%; and SJM valve: 1 or 2%).

Late survival

There were 16 deaths in the 534 patients followed-up, resulting in a late mortality of 2.8% and a relative survival of 97.2%. Causes of death in the 16 patients were: heart failure (n=6); cerebral hemorrhage (n=4); cerebral thromboembolism (n=1); prosthetic valve endocarditis (n=1); unknown (possible arrhythmia) (n=4).

Thrombogenicity and thromboembolic events

Thromboembolism is a very important problem, and one which is still not completely resolved in patients with cardiac valve prostheses. We found 6 cases of thromboembolism out of 534 followed patients with SJM valves in aortic, mitral and mitral/aortic positions (Table 2). Out of 534 patients followed-up, 6 thromboembolic events were 1.12% of the total number of patients operated on with SJM valves in aortic, mitral and mitral/aortic positions. The overall thromboembolic rate was 0.48% per patient year. Of the 6 patients having thromboembolic events, 3 (50%) followed a correct anticoagulation therapy and 3 (50%) did not. The thromboembolic rate of 1.12% we found in patients with SJM prostheses is very low and decidedly less than the thromboembolic rate for patients with unoperated valvular disease.

All patients with a SJM prosthesis followed a correct anticoagulation therapy with acenocoumarol (Sintrom®) (except the 3 cited above) to maintain a prothrombin level of 20–30% of normal.

We recommend this regimen even though we believe a patient with a SJM valve in sinus rhythm can suspend anticoagulation therapy for relatively long periods of time without particular disadvantage.

Chronic intravascular hemolysis and flow characteristics

Initial postoperative data on patients with the SJM prosthesis showed bilirubinemia and haptoglobinemia levels to be within the normal limits or slightly lower than the norm, but without clinical symptoms or laboratory signs of anemia. Patients with symptoms of anemia or hemolysis almost always have abnormal flow characteristics with turbulent flow (9) due to paravalvular leaks, or other pathological processes, such as sepsis.

Prosthetic noise

Prosthetic noise was not perceived by the SJM patients who 3–6 months postoperatively had adapted to their mechanical prosthesis, and were able to live a normal life without exhibiting an inferiority complex when compared to the healthy public.

The SJM mechanical prosthesis – valve of choice for routine heart valve replacement

For several reasons, we prefer the mechanical SJM bileaflet prosthesis which we have been using for 6 years (10, 11). This valve has excellent hemodynamics in small sizes (4, 12–16), particularly when used according to our formula which correlates valve orifice diameter to body surface area. Since the use of this formula and the valve, aortoplasty enlargement has become unusual for us. The low profile valve can be implanted without obstructing the left ventricular outflow tract when the valve is used in the mitral position. This low profile is the reason we use the valve in almost all double implants. Implantations are simpler with this valve in comparison with bioprostheses in which, at times, a stent has ruptured the left ventricular wall.

The SJM valve has shown a low incidence of thromboembolism (13, 17, 18) which allows the possibility of suspending anticoagulant therapy for long periods of time as well as during the first 2–3 months of pregnancy. There has been an absence of clinical hemolysis with no clinical signs of anemia (9), and the low noise level of the prosthesis has been well tolerated by patients. Phonocardiography (19), M-mode and two-dimensional echocardiography (19, 20) and cinefluoroscopy (21) have proved to be reliable noninvasive techniques for the long-term follow-up of the SJM prostheses.

We use bioprostheses in the following circumstances:

1. single valve implants in patients over 60 years old who have large valvular orifices;
2. patients who cannot tolerate anticoagulant therapy because of diseases predisposing to bleeding;
3. patients who do not want to submit to the constant laboratory control which anticoagulation requires;
4. patients who do not accept the noise of a mechanical valve;
5. fertile women who desire children without risk to the fetus or risk of hemorrhage to the mother. These women are informed that during pregnancy the bioprosthesis may have precocious calcification and infective prosthetic valve endocarditis during the puerperal period.

References

1. Roberts WC (1976) Choosing a substitute cardiac valve: type, size, surgeon. Ann J Cardiol 38:633
2. Emery RW, Nicoloff DM (1979) St. Jude Medical cardiac valve prosthesis. In vitro studies. J Thorac Cardiovasc Surg 78:269
3. Scotten NL, Racca RG, Nugent AH et al (1981) New tilting disc cardiac valve prostheses. J Thorac Cardiovasc Surg 82:136

4. Horstkotte D, Haerten K, Seipel L et al (1983) Central hemodynamics at rest and during exercise after mitral valve replacement with different prostheses. Circulation 68 (Suppl II): 161
5. Bruss KH, Reul H, van Gilse J et al (1983) Pressure drops and velocity fields at four mechanical heart valve prostheses: Björk-Shiley Standard, Björk-Shiley convex-concave, Hall-Kaster, and St. Jude Medical. Life Supp Syst 1:3
6. Konno S, Imai Y, Iida Y et al (1975) A new method for prosthetic valve replacement in congenital aortic stenosis associated with hypoplasia of the aortic ring. J Thorac Cardiovasc Surg 70:909
7. New York Heart Association (1964) The Criteria Committee of the New York Heart Association: Diseases of Heart and Blood Vessels (nomenclature and criteria of diagnosis), 6th ed. Little, Brown and Co, Boston
8. Horstkotte D, Haerten K, Schulte HD et al (1983) Hemodynamical findings at rest and during exercise after implantation of different mitral valve prostheses with equal tissue annulus diameters. Z Kardiol 72:385
9. Horstkotte D, Aul C, Seipel L et al (1983) Influence of valve type and valve function on chronic intravascular hemolysis following mitral and aortic valve replacement using alloprostheses. Z Kardiol 72:119
10. D'Alessandro LC (1981) St. Jude Medical prosthesis: Clinical results. Second International Symposium, San Diego
11. D'Alessandro LC, Baruffi E, Giordano F et al (1983) Italian experience with the St. Jude Medical valve. In: DeBakey ME (ed) Advances in Cardiac Valves. Yorke Medical Books, New York p 41
12. Emery RW, Anderson RW, Lindsay WG et al (1979) Clinical and hemodynamic results with the St. Jude Medical aortic valve prosthesis. Surg Forum 30:235
13. Horstkotte D, Haerten K, Herzer JA et al (1981) Preliminary clinical and hemodynamic results after mitral valve replacement using St. Jude Medical prostheses in comparison with the Björk-Shiley valve. J Thorac Cardiovasc Surg 29:93
14. Gill CC, King HC, Lytle BW et al (1982) Early clinical evaluation after aortic valve replacement with the St. Jude Medical valve in patients with a small aortic root. Circulation 66 (Part II):147
15. Nicoloff DM, Emery RW, Arom KV et al (1981) Clinical and hemodynamic results with the St. Jude Medical cardiac valve prosthesis. A three-year experience. J Thorac Cardiovasc Surg 82:674
16. Wortham DC, Tri TB, Bowen TE (1981) Hemodynamic evaluation of the St. Jude Medical valve prosthesis in the small aortic anulus. J Thorac Cardiovasc Surg 81:61
17. Hunt D, Sloman G, Sutton L (1981) The St. Jude Medical valve: The Australian experience. Med J Aust 2:276
18. Lillehei C (1982) Worldwide experience with the St. Jude Medical valve prosthesis: Clinical and hemodynamic results. Cardiovasc Med 1:309
19. Chaux A, Gray RJ, Matloff JM et al (1981) An appreciation of the new St. Jude valvular prosthesis. J Thorac Cardiovasc Surg 81:202
20. Garcia-Fernandez MA, Actigao R, Banuelos F et al (1982) M-mode and 2-dimensional echocardiography of the St. Jude prosthesis. Rev Esp Cardio 35:123
21. Castaneda ZW, Nicoloff DM, Jorgensen C et al (1980) In vivo radiographic appearance of the St. Jude valve prosthesis. Radiology 134:775

Authors' address:

Luigi C. D'Alessandro, M. D.
Cardiac Surgery Department
S. Camillo Hospital
Rome
Italy

The Choice Between Valve Preservation and Valve Replacement

N. G. De Vega

Before open-heart techniques were developed, surgeons could only direct their efforts toward achieving repair of diseased valves. Surprisingly, certain techniques developed then are still the basis for surgical procedures used today.

Since 1957, when open-heart techniques became widespread, and 1961, when the first artificial valve became commercially available, surgeons on both sides of the Atlantic have been attempting repair for all types of valvular dysfunctions. Such techniques as Kay's (1) and Wooler's (2) annuloplasties became known and were used by many surgeons working in this field. Since then, surgeons have been faced with the dilemma of valvular repair versus valvular replacement. The choice has been cyclically influenced by the type of disease pathology, available prostheses and the improvement of conservative techniques.

In the beginning, most valvular lesions were caused by rheumatic endocarditis and most patients were young people with flexible, noncalcified valves. Later, due to the decrease of rheumatic fever in well-developed countries, the number of calcified valves defying repair increased progressively (3). Furthermore, new lesions involving the mitral valve, such as prolapse, with and without mitral valve insufficiency (4) have been described and a better understanding of ischemic involvement of the atrioventricular valves (5) has renewed interest in valvuloplasties.

Development of valve repair and valve replacement techniques

Over the last 25 years, dozens of new valve models with theoretical advantages over former valves have been designed and commercially launched. But the supposed advantages were not always demonstrated over time, when the valves were used clinically. In the early '70s, as a result of the work of different groups such as Ionescu, Binet, Ross, Carpentier and others, the first bioprostheses were manufactured and distributed by Hancock. At that time a considerable number of mitral valvulopathies, which until then had been considered suitable for repair, began to be treated with replacement using a porcine xenograft. Five to six years later, when the limitations and contraindications of these valve replacements became apparent (6,7), the emphasis was again put back upon valve repair.

Concurrent with this evolution of mechanical and biological valves, different techniques for valve repair were described (Table 1) which improved the short- and long-term results of these procedures. Many of these procedures are known by the name of the surgeon who developed them. In an attempt to clarify their diverse characteristics (see Figures 1–4), we have classified them into four main groups.

Besides these techniques, the works of McGoon (8) and Carpentier (9) should be mentioned because their accomplishments in the repair of leaflets and chordae tendineae have broadened the indications and improved the results of conservative valve surgery. In an analysis of valvuloplasty, the mitral, aortic and tricuspid valves must be clearly separated

Table 1. Classification of the annuloplasties

A. Reduction of the annulus without support
B. Annular reduction supported by sutures
C. Selective reduction supported by strips or pledgets of synthetic material
D. Annular reduction by different types of rings

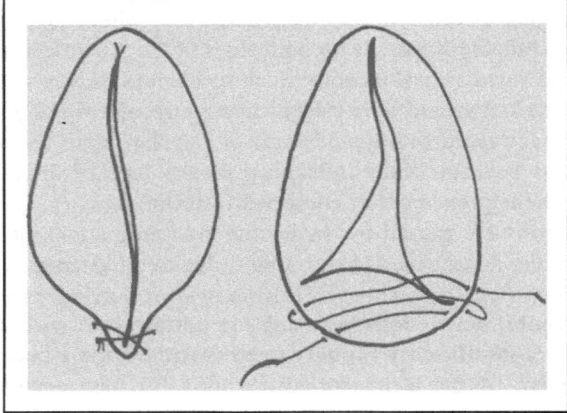

Fig. 1. Reduction of the annulus of an atrioventricular valve without support (annuloplasties type A)

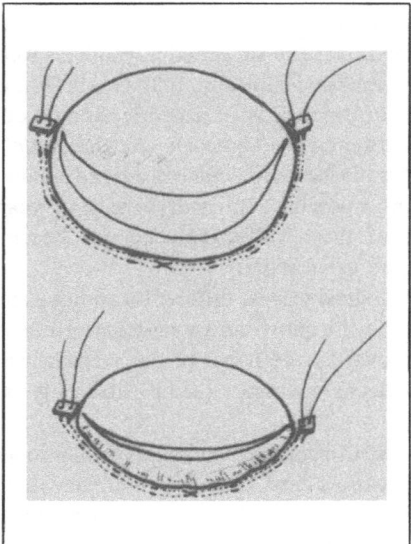

Fig. 2. Annular or semi-annular reduction of an insufficient atrioventricular valve supported by sutures (annuloplasties type B)

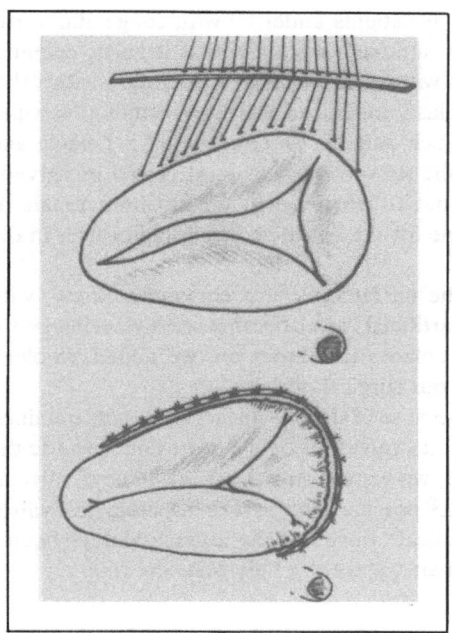

Fig. 3. Selective reduction supported by strips or pledgets of synthetic material (annuloplasties type C)

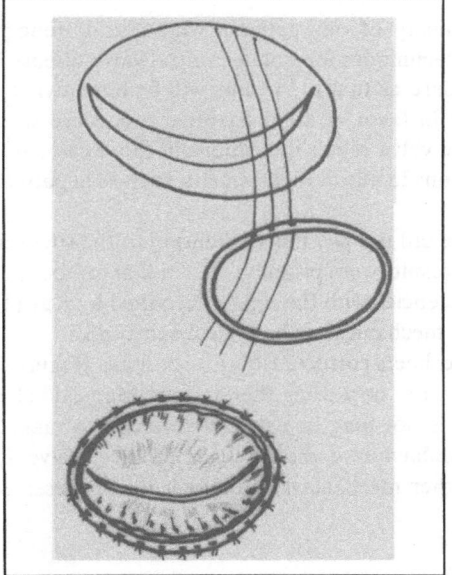

Fig. 4. Annular reduction by different types of rings (annuloplasties type D)

since their anatomical characteristics, hemodynamic conditions and the pathology affecting them make it impossible to analyse them as a whole.

The decision to treat valvulopathies by repair or replacement depends on patient-related factors and the anatomical characteristics of the valve to be treated. In some cases we consider repair compulsory, while in others repair should be done only if the surgical findings favour such a decision. For example, in patients under 20 with congenital aortic stenosis, we rarely consider valve replacement, although we know that if aortic commissurotomy is performed, most of these patients will require a second operation with valve replacement later in life. We consider valvuloplasty instead of the more common valvular replacement for a combined mitral lesion in which only the anterior leaflet is flexible and pliable, the commissures are not calcified and the subvalvular apparatus is well preserved. Before attempting to answer the query of what to do when in doubt about repair or replacement, a description of what we have done for the mitral and tricuspid orifices in the last 25 years is necessary.

Until 1961, the only procedure we used on the mitral valve was commissurotomy, with mostly closed techniques. Later, when the first artificial valves became readily available, we combined mitral commissurotomy and valve replacement. Later on, we added Wooler's repair (2) and the Alvarez mitral prosthesis to our surgical practice.

In 1969, we switched to fascia lata valves (10) because of the unsatisfactory results obtained with the Alvarez prosthesis; but we used fascia lata valves for only a short time because the outcome was less than satisfactory (11). In 1971, we began using the Björk-Shiley® valve as our mechanical valve of choice and the Hancock® porcine xenograft as our biological valve. Since 1980 we have been using the St. Jude Medical® valve and the Ionescu-Shiley® bovine xenograft for valve replacements. For valve repair we use the Puiy-Massana ring.

Mitral and tricuspid repair operations

Mitral commissurotomy is still indicated in many of our patients with mitral stenosis. However, we advocate the use of conservative techniques for isolated mitral valve disease in those patients whose anatomical conditions assure us that the results will be hemodynamically satisfactory and long-lasting. We are not in favor of a conservative procedure when another valve must be replaced. We extend the valve repair indications in those cases with less suitable anatomy and formal contraindications to mitral replacement, such as in patients under 18 years of age.

At the beginning of our surgical experience, we did not pay much attention to the tricuspid valve. When we realized that some of our poor results were probably due to that attitude, we began correcting some of the tricuspid incompetencies with the repair described by Kay (1). In other instances, we replaced the valve with mechanical or biological substitutes.

Since 1972, 95% of the tricuspid lesions have been corrected by a technique (Figure 5) described by us (12). If repair is impossible, we are now using the St. Jude Medical valve. Although our experience with this prosthesis is not long or extensive enough to make a definitive statement, our feeling is that the behavior of the St. Jude Medical valve for tricuspid replacement is better than that of other mechanical or biological prostheses we previously used.

Valve preservation or valve replacement? What to do when in doubt

Now we arrive at the question of what should be done when deciding whether to preserve or replace the valve. Our response is clear-cut: waste little time in doubting! Doubts will result in long ischemic time, less than optimal myocardial protection and potentially harmful extensions of the cardiopulmonary bypass.

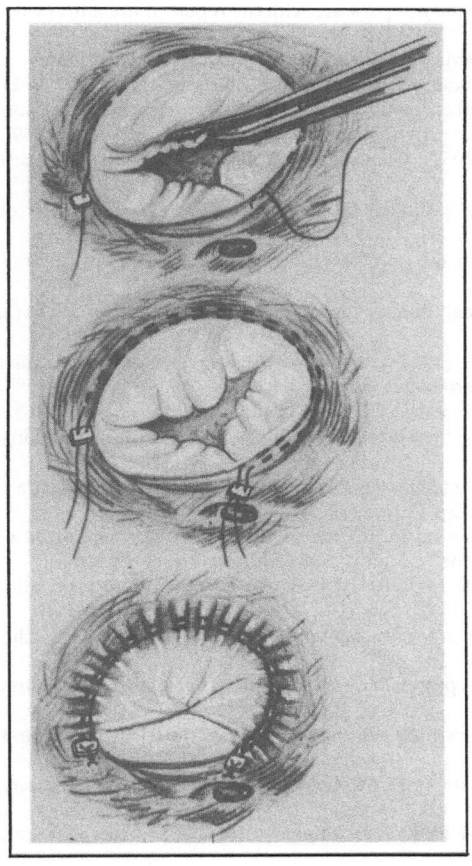

Fig. 5. Annuloplasty of tricuspid valves in the technique of De Vega

In our opinion, when you are not sure that mitral repair will result in a satisfactory anatomical and hemodynamic outcome (2, 8, 9, 13–16), a prompt replacement with a mechanical or biological prosthesis is the best solution.

We very seldom decide to replace the tricuspid valve (17) since we think that any replacement of this valve would yield worse long-term results than those achieved by repair (1, 18–20) even if the resulting valve function turned out to be imperfect. A thorough survey of the literature shows diverse findings after valve replacement (21–24) and valve reconstruction (13–15, 18, 25, 26) and contradictory opinions by outstanding groups. This might be due to poor statistical analysis, or to different pathologies.

To the following questions the answers are still uncertain: Is the Wooler annuloplasty (2) still a valid technique for correction of mitral incompetence? Which is the best choice when tricuspid replacement is needed – mechanical or biological? Should mitral incompetence caused by rupture of the anterior leaflet chordae be repaired?

References

1. Peterffy A, Jonasson R, Szamosi A et al (1980) Comparison of Kay's and De Vega's annuloplasty in surgical treatment of tricuspid incompetence. Scand J Cardiovasc Surg 14:249

2. Wooler GH, Nixon PGF, Grimshaw VA et al (1962) Experience with the repair of the mitral valve in mitral incompetence. Thorax 17:49
3. Loogen F, Horstkotte D (1982) Therapy of cardiovascular disease – Valvular heart disease. In: Bleifeld W, Mathey D (eds) Therapy of cardiovascular disease. Thieme, Stuttgart – New York, p 21
4. Kay JH, Krohn BG, Zubiate et al (1979) Surgical correction of severe mitral valve prolapse without mitral insufficiency but with pronounced cardiac arrhythmias. J Thorac Cardiovasc Surg 78:259
5. Burch GE, de Pasquale NP, Phillips JH (1962) Clinical manifestation of papillary muscle dysfunction. Arch Intern Med 112:112
6. Fishbein MC, Giessen SA, Collins JJ (1977) Pathology in patients with glutaraldehyde-fixed porcine cardiac valves. Am J Cardiol 40:331
7. Geha AS, Laks H, Stansel HC et al (1979) Late failure of porcine valve heterografts in children. J Thorac Cardiovasc Surg 78:351
8. McGoon D (1959) Repair of mitral insufficiency due to ruptured chordae tendineae. J Thorac Cardiovasc Surg 39:357–362
9. Capentier A, Cauvaud S, Fabiani JN et al (1980) Reconstructive surgery of mitral valve incompetence: Ten-year appraisal. J Thorac Cardiovasc Surg 79:338
10. Senning A (1967) Fascia lata replacement of the aortic valve. J Thorac Cardiovasc Surg 54:465
11. Senning A, Rothlin M (1973) Reconstruction of the aortic valve with fascia lata: Initial and long-term results. Vasc Surg 7:29
12. De Vega NG (1972) La anuloplastia selectiva, regulable y permanente: una tècnica original para el tratamiento de la insuficiencia tricúspide. Rev Esp Cardiol 25:555
13. Durán CG (1980) Conservative operation for mitral insufficiency: Critical analysis supported by postoperative hemodynamic studies of 72 patients. J Thorac and Cardiovasc Surg 79:326
14. Shore DF, Wong P, Paneth M (1980) Results of mitral valvuloplasty with a suture plication technique. J Thorac Cardiovasc Surg 79:349
15. Adebo DA et al (1983) Conservative surgery for mitral valve disease: Clinical and echo-cardiographic analysis of results. Thorax 38:564
16. Frater RW, Gabbay S, Shore D et al (1983) Reproducible replacement of elongated or ruptured mitral valve chordae. Ann Thorac Surg 35:14
17. Mestres CA, Igual A, Murtra M (1983) The Björk-Shiley tilting disc valve in the tricuspid position. Scand J Thorac Cardiovasc Surg 17:197
18. Charlesworth DC et al (1983) Assessment of mitral and tricuspid competence after valvuloplasty. Ann Thorac Surg 35:105
19. Brugger JJ, Egloff L, Rothlin M et al (1982) Tricuspidal annuloplasty: Results and complications. Thorac Cardiovasc Surgeon 30:284
20. Haerten K, Seipel L, Loogen F et al (1978) Hemodynamic studies after De Vega's tricuspid annuloplasty. Circulation 58 (Suppl I):28
21. Starr A, Edwards ML (1961) Mitral replacement: Clinical experience with a ball-valve prosthesis. Ann Surg 154:726
22. Tepley JF, Grunkemeier GL, Sutherland DH et al (1981) The ultimate prognosis after valve replacement: An assessment at twenty years. Ann Thorac Surg 32:111
23. Bonchek LI (1981) Cardiac valve replacement. Ann Thorac Surg 32:editorial
24. Horstkotte D, Haerten K, Herzer JA et al (1983) Five-years results after randomized mitral valve replacement with Björk-Shiley, Lillehei-Kaster and Starr-Edwards prostheses. Thorac Cardiovasc Surg 31:206
25. Reed GE, Pooley RW, Maggio RA (1980) Durability of measured mitral annuloplasty: Seventeen-year study. J Thorac Cardiovasc Surg 79:321
26. de Caleya D, Sarnago F, Galinanes M et al (1983) Fracture of Carpentier's ring in a patient with tricuspid annuloplasty. Thorac Cardiovasc Surg 31:175

Author's address:
N. G. de Vega, M. D.
Hospital Regional Carlos Haya
Málaga
Spain

The Limits of Central Hemodynamic Improvement by Heart Valve Replacement

D. Horstkotte and J. Delaye

Besides the specific complications accompanying prosthetic heart valve replacement, its success is substantially dependent on two conditions: first on the valve function and second on the question of whether and to what degree the impaired left ventricular function is normalized postoperatively. Only the restitution of the valve function can be influenced directly by prosthetic heart valve replacement. With chronic valvular lesions, however, in the overwhelming majority of cases, a restitution of physiological hemodynamic properties is not possible (1). This is caused by the fact that the space needed for sewing ring and valve poppet represents an obstruction of the blood flow, conditioning a higher transprosthetic pressure gradient the more the valve orifice area is narrowed (1,2). The hemodynamic properties of the prosthesis therefore become more unfavourable with the lowering of the relation between effective and total valve orifice area. Changes of flow profiles at artificial heart valves, concomitant with increasing pressure gradients, result in higher turbulences, as well as other effects. The consecutive traumatization of formed blood elements can – besides hemolysis – also initiate a release of thrombocyte-specific enzymes and aggregation of platelets.

The degree of blood stream obstruction by artificial valves is mainly determined by two of their construction principles: on the one hand the size of the sewing ring, that means the relation between outer and inner diameter of the valve must be regarded. On the other hand the narrowing of the valve orifice by the occluder is of importance. One has to bear in mind that not all occluders of mechanical prostheses and not all leaflets of bioprostheses reach that degree of opening, which can be documented in in vitro tests (1,3).

Consequently, some of the heart valve prostheses developed earlier presented negative clinical results corresponding to an incomplete opening of the disc (3,4). Therefore, reliable comparative studies of pressure-flow relations of prosthetic heart valves require invasive re-studies of operated patients.

Hemodynamic studies at rest and under exercise are of importance especially after mitral and tricuspid valve replacement, because the transprosthetic gradients cause more distinctly negative effects after replacement of atrio-ventricular valves than after aortic valve replacement. After mitral valve replacement, in relation to the type of prosthesis and the duration of the disease, a more or less extensive normalization of the pressure values in the pulmonary circulation can be expected at rest. The gradual postoperative decrease of pulmonary artery pressure in some cases, however, can take more than one year. For the duration of this process, it is somewhat decisive that the "statics" of the left ventricle and its geometry is markedly altered by the resection of the mitral valve, including chordae tendiniae and the tips of the papillary muscles. Hence, it is understandable that echocardio-graphic studies starting early after prosthetic heart valve replacement and continued up to one year after operation in mitral lesions patients documented an early postoperative impairment of the left ventricular function.

Corresponding to the valve type and the persistent flow obstruction into the left ventricle, the decrease of pressures in pulmonary circulation after mitral valve replacement is more or less expressed. With those mechanical or biological valves developed recently, an extended normalization of the pulmonary artery pressure could be achieved. Nevertheless, the improvement after prosthetic valve replacement following chronic mitral valve lesions usually amounts to only one degree according to the New York Heart Association's classification (5,6). This is the result of the postoperatively resistant pathological increase of pressures in the pulmonary circulation under exercise. Besides the pressure gradient persisting after valve implantation, transprosthetic regurgitations also may gain in hemodynamic importance.

The volume loss of an artificial valve consists of the closing volume and the leakage flow. The closing volume is that volume which is regurged until the complete closure of the valve occluder. The leakage flow is the volume regurged due to the constructional properties of the prosthesis when closed. Such regurgitation volumes are willingly tolerated to achieve a certain blood flow through the closed valve at places where the flow velocities are low with the normal blood flows, so that platelet aggregation or platelet adhesion is reduced.

More than after mitral valve replacement, the success of a prosthetic aortic valve replacement is also dependent on how far the left ventricular function, which had been impaired more or less preoperatively, is normalized (7). If functional impairment of the left ventricle is mainly a consequence of a pressure and volume load, an extended restoration can be expected after operation. If, however, myocardial damage with irreversible contractility impairment is dominating, even after restoration of the valve function, the clinical outcome may be unsatisfactory because of the persistent myocardial failure. The pressure and volume load existing with aortic valve disease leads to an increase of pre- and after-load with hypertrophy and, corresponding to the degree of valve incompetence, to a dilatation of the left ventricle, so that the left ventricular end-diastolic pressure and the end-systolic volume increase, while stroke volume and ejection fraction decrease.

The postoperative hemodynamic improvement in patients with aortic valve replacement is manifested in a normalization of the cardiac index, stroke volume index and ejection fraction as well as in left ventricular end-diastolic pressure and the corresponding pressures in the pulmonary artery and the left atrium (8).

The hemodynamic quality of a prosthesis can be extensively characterized by the transprosthetic gradient and the volume loss. Hemodynamic advantages of a type of prosthesis, however, have to be correlated to the complications it induces. Accordingly, sometimes hemodynamic disadvantages, e. g., increased leakage flow through the prosthesis, are accepted to reduce the risk of thrombus formation near the valve housing.

Prosthetic aortic valve replacement is very exacting to the hemodynamic properties of a prosthesis, if only valves of small sizes can be implanted: valve and sewing ring require a space dependent on the construction of a certain prosthesis model, so that the relation between outer and inner valve diameter becomes an important parameter of the hemodynamic properties of the prosthesis. Because of their larger sewing rings xenografts or ball prostheses present disadvantages. Unsatisfactory hemodynamic results, especially after implantation of small xenografts in aortic positions, are well known. Therefore, the proposal has already been made to implant small xenografts only in patients with a body surface area of less than 1.8 m^2 (9).

References

1. Horstkotte D, Haerten K, Seipel L et al (1982) Central hemodynamics at rest and during exercise after mitral valve replacement with different prostheses. Circulation 68 (Suppl II):161
2. Horstkotte D, Schulte HD, Körfer R et al (1982) Mitral valve replacement using different prosthetic valves. Int J Artif Organs 5:177
3. Sigwart U, Schmidt H, Gleichmann U et al (1976) In vivo evaluation of the Lillehei-Kaster heart valve prosthesis. Ann Thorac Surg 22:213
4. Ohlmeier H, Mannebach H, Greitemeier A (1982) Clinical follow-up of patients after valve replacement with Omniscience cardiac valves: Can this valve be recommended? Z Kardiol 71:350
5. Horstkotte D, Haerten K, Herzer JA et al (1983) Five-year results after randomized mitral valve replacement with Björk-Shiley, Lillehei-Kaster, and Starr-Edwards prostheses. Thorac Cardiovasc Surg 31:206
6. Haerten K, Horstkotte D (1982) The influence of operative procedures on the long-term follow-up and the prognosis of mitral valve disease. Herz/Kreisl 9:475
7. Schwarz F, Flameng W, Thormann J et al (1978) Recovery from myocardial failure after aortic valve replacement. Am J Cardiol 45:854
8. Horstkotte D, Haerten K, Körfer R et al (1983) Hemodynamic findings at rest and during exercise after implantation of different aortic valve prostheses. Z Kardiol 72:429
9. DiSesa VJ, Collins JJ, Cohn LH (1982) Valve replacement in the small aortic anulus aorta: performance of the Hancock modified-orifice bioprosthesis In: Cohn LH, Gallucci (eds) Cardiac Bioprostheses. Yorke, New York, p 552

Authors' address:

Dr. Dieter Horstkotte
Medizinische Klinik der
Universität Düsseldorf
Moorenstraße 5
4000 Düsseldorf
F.R.G.

Can the Hemodynamics of Prosthetic Heart Valves be Evaluated Sufficiently by In Vitro Tests?

M. Gottwik, S. Hartung, O. Epe, S. Langsdorf, J. Thormann and M. Schlepper

Four tilting disc prostheses and one bileaflet valve are currently available for implantation in the aortic position. At the time of their clinical trials, few comparative clinical data were available, and rarely could in vitro data, obtained under identical testing conditions, be supplied for competitive valves (1–8). In vitro results of different valve types, however, can only be compared when obtained by the same testing procedure and testing apparatus.

Since each pulse duplicator has indigenous qualities that may influence results, pressure/flow relationships of one valve cannot necessarily be compared to the pressure/flow values for another valve obtained in a different pulse duplicator (6). Therefore, in vitro results of different valves taken under different testing procedures can only be compared if exact knowledge of the testing procedure and testing apparatus has been obtained and adjustments made accordingly. A more convincing alternative to correcting for the idiosyncrasies of any testing procedure would be to test several valves under identical conditions. Therefore, we developed a pulse duplicator to test and compare the mechanical properties of new valves (9).

A differentiation between tissue anulus size and effective orifice area is necessary because any prosthetic orifice ring will produce some obstruction of the outflow track. The valve's profile and the bulk of the suture ring influence the pressure drop across a valve (10). The valve's design influences hemodynamics via the opening angle of the occluder(s), the velocity and friction of blood flow during occluder motion and the amount of backflow during closure (3, 8, 11–13).

Pulse duplicator studies on five mechanical aortic prostheses

Four tilting disc and one bileaflet aortic valve with an internal diameter of approximately 20 mm were selected for this study. Björk-Shiley® Spherical, Björk-Shiley® Convexo-Concave, Medtronic Hall®, Omniscience® and St. Jude Medical® bileaflet valves were tested under identical conditions in a pulse duplicator that was developed in our laboratory and has been described earlier (9). All valves were fitted into an outflow track of 23 mm diameter to equalize differences in width of the valvular cage and suture ring.

Pressures were recorded in the left ventricle and in the aorta 5 cm downstream from the aortic valve. Pressure gradients between the left ventricle and the aorta were differentiated automatically and recorded by simultaneous recording.

Electromagnetic flowmeter measurements were recorded on the same tracing and gradients determined at the point of maximum flow 4 cm downstream from the aortic valve. Flow recordings were not used for determination of cardiac output. They were used as an indicator of backflow in relative units, as percent of stroke volume, and they were obtained by comparative planimetry of the area under the 'zero-line' during forward and backward flow. Cardiac output was determined by direct measurement. The exact cycle length was measured by the use of time markers on the recording. Pressure transducers (Gould-Statham P23ID) were connected to an Electronics for Medicine VR8 amplifier-recorder unit. All records were obtained on photographic paper with a UV light recorder at a paper speed of 75 mm/sec.

Identical machine settings were chosen for the testing of all valves. Displaced volume was slightly decreased with the frequency increase because air was used for expansion of rubber membranes to transmit the pump function to the ventricle (Table 1). The baseline-systolic

Table 1. Synopsis of all measurement points and calculated values appearing in Figs. 1–4

Valve	Frequency bpm	Flow ml	PAO mm Hg	PLV mm Hg	GRAD mm Hg	SV ml	GR/SV mm Hg/ml	Valve area cm²
Björk	56.2	4480	148.0	166.0	18.5	79.6	.23	1.32
Shiley	68.7	5230	152.0	183.5	31.5	76.0	.41	1.13
Standard	84.1	5850	156.0	107.5	51.5	69.5	.74	0.96
	93.8	6530	157.0	224.0	67.5	69.6	.96	0.94
	207.8	7320	155.5	236.5	81.0	67.8	1.19	0.91
	123.5	8140	155.0	243.0	88.0	65.9	1.33	0.95
Björk	54.6	4580	136.0	158.5	22.5	83.8	.26	1.17
Shiley	67.7	5530	141.0	178.5	37.5	81.6	.45	1.03
Convexo-	78.7	6100	144.5	196.5	52.0	72.5	.67	0.97
Concave	91.9	7067	144.5	208.5	64.0	76.8	.83	0.98
	104.0	8087	143.5	218.0	74.5	77.7	.95	0.99
	121.3	8800	142.0	226.0	84.5	72.5	1.15	1.00
Medtronic	54.3	4700	134.5	153.0	18.5	86.5	.21	1.36
Hall	67.2	5590	140.0	171.0	31.0	83.1	.37	1.21
	79.0	6453	143.5	192.0	48.5	81.6	.59	1.10
	93.4	7280	143.5	204.0	60.5	77.8	.76	1.03
	104.4	8500	143.5	221.0	77.5	79.8	.97	1.03
	121.8	9420	146.0	233.0	87.0	77.3	1.12	1.04
Omni-	55.2	4720	138.0	160.0	22.0	85.4	.25	1.28
science	68.2	5773	142.0	176.0	34.0	84.5	.40	1.16
	80.1	6360	147.0	196.0	49.0	79.3	.61	1.04
	92.7	7373	145.0	211.0	66.0	79.5	.83	1.05
	106.0	8040	144.0	220.0	76.0	75.8	1.00	1.01
	119.6	9100	146.0	229.0	83.0	76.0	1.09	1.05
St. Jude	55.0	4880	138.0	156.5	18.5	88.6	.20	1.47
Medical	67.8	5770	147.0	179.5	32.5	85.0	.38	1.18
	80.1	6427	149.5	196.0	46.5	80.1	.58	1.08
	92.2	7453	148.5	210.0	61.5	80.7	.76	1.06
	106.8	8446	147.0	216.5	69.5	79.0	.86	1.07
	118.3	9340	148.0	228.0	80.0	78.9	1.01	1.11

PAO = Aortic pressure
PLV = Left ventricular pressure
GRAD = Gradient
SV = Stroke volume
GR/SV = Gradient/stroke volume

left ventricular pressure was adjusted to 140 mm Hg by variation of peripheral resistance for each valvular model.

The valvular function for all five valves is shown over a range of frequencies from 54 to 124 bpm (Table 1) resulting in an increase of cardiac output from 4.5 l to 9.4 l. A nearly linear increase in cardiac output is shown in Figure 1. The incline of the single curves indicates the mechanical function of a prosthesis at higher frequencies. All more modern valves performed at a comparable level; for example, the Björk-Shiley Spherical valve showed a decline of cardiac output with higher frequencies.

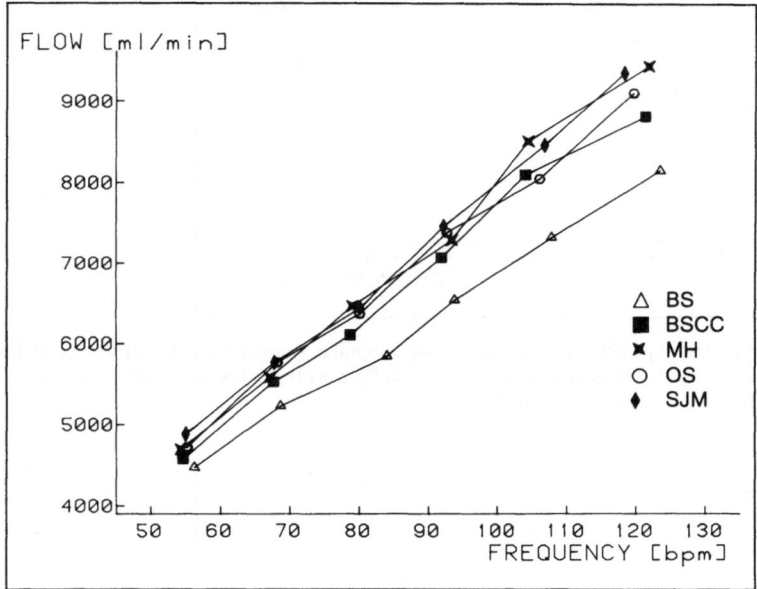

Fig. 1. Frequency is plotted against flow, indicating a close to linear relationship of cardiac output and frequency. Values see Table 1.

△ Björk Shiley Standard (BS)
■ Björk Shiley Convexo-Concave (BSCC)
✚ Medtronic Hall (MH)
○ Omniscience (OS)
◆ St. Jude Medical (SJM)

The stroke volume provided by our pulse duplicator decreased slightly in a linear fashion because of increased friction in the pulse duplicator system during gas exchange (Table 1). This effect, however, is augmented by an increased resistance against displaced volume generated by the individual valves.

Again, the Björk-Shiley Spherical valve showed the largest decrease of stroke volume, whereas the other valves are in a close range. The decrease of stroke volume for all valves amounted to approximately 10% across the entire range of frequencies tested.

The loss of pressure across a valve during simultaneous measurement of left ventricular and aortic pressures is frequently referred to when valves are tested in experimental settings. The pressure gradient of all five valves at maximal systolic flow is shown in Figure 2 (Table 1) as determined at six different frequencies.

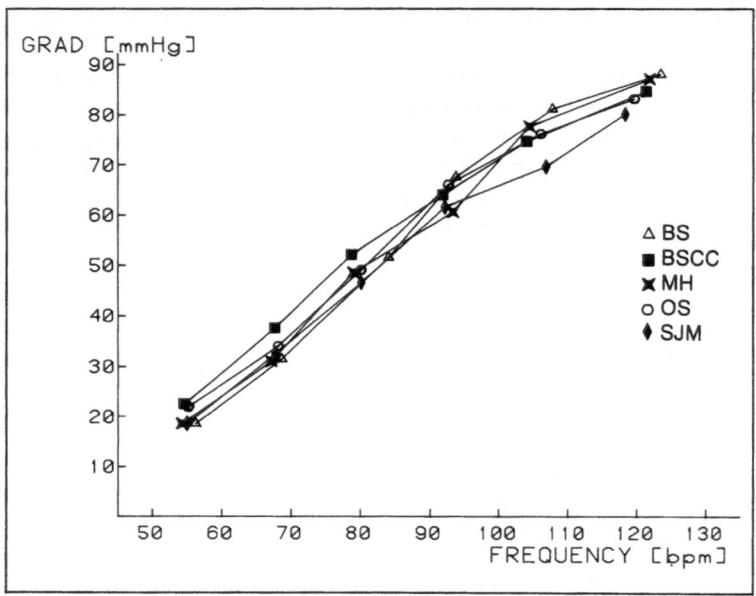

Fig. 2. Frequency is plotted against gradient, indicating a similar performance of all valves at low frequencies. Differences are shown at frequencies above 80 bpm with △ (BS), exhibiting the highest, ♦ (SJM) the lowest gradient (values see Table 1).

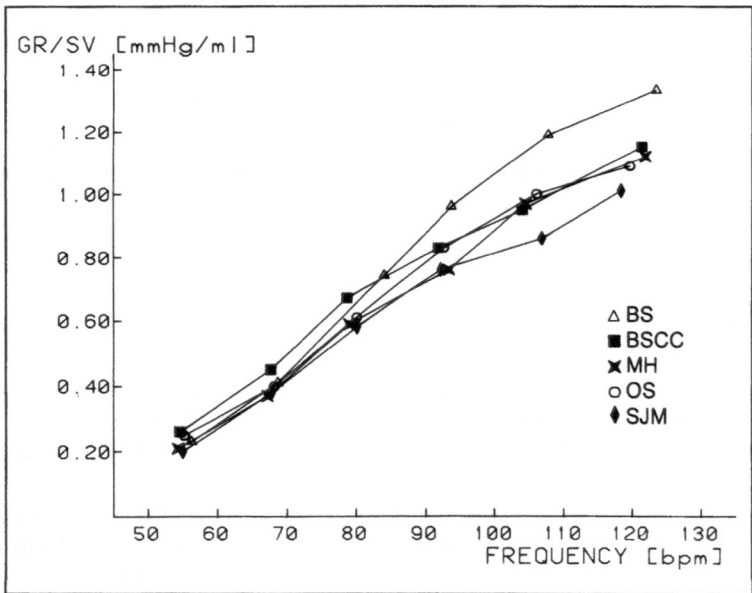

Fig. 3. Frequency (bpm) is plotted against gradient/stroke volume (mm Hg/ml) (values see Table 1). ♦ (SJM) shows the overall best performance; △ (BS) performs poorly at high frequencies; ✚ (MH), O (OS), ■ (BSCC) are similar at high frequencies, whereas ■ (BSCC) performs poorly at low frequencies.

The gradient was found to be almost linear over the tested range for all valves, and the St. Jude Medical bileaflet valve produced the lowest gradient at frequencies above 70 bpm. To consider flow, frequency and valvular stenosis expressed as pressure drop across the valve, the gradient (mm Hg) was divided by the stroke volume (ml) and plotted against frequency (see Figure 3 and Table 1). At frequencies below 70 bpm, the valvular performance was comparable for all models. Above 80 bpm, a progressive separation of the valves became obvious. The Björk-Shiley Spherical valve clearly fell off at high frequencies and the St. Jude Medical prosthesis showed the best overall performance. The remaining three models did not show major differences.

The Gorlin formula (14) was used to determine the effective orifice area. The results are shown in Figure 4 and Table 1. A steep decrease of the calculated effective orifice area occurred during increasing heart rate for all valves because of decreasing stroke volume and increasing gradient at higher frequencies. The Gorlin formula clearly separated the calculated effective orifice areas of the valves. At frequencies above 80 bpm, the Björk-Shiley Spherical valve showed the poorest performance, followed by Björk-Shiley Convexo-Concave, Omniscience and Medtronic Hall prostheses. The St. Jude Medical bileaflet valve had the largest effective orifice area.

Regurgitation during valvular closure is another parameter of valvular function. The closing volume for each valve was determined by planimetry of the flowmeter tracings and given as

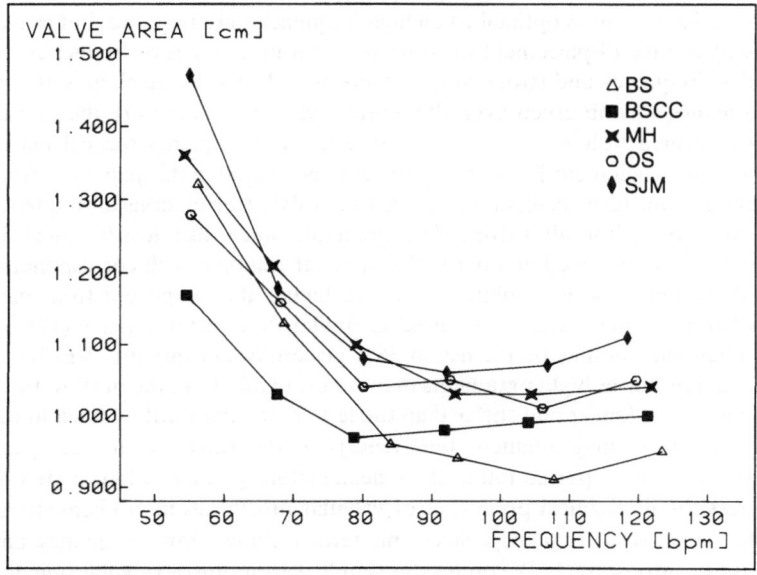

Fig. 4. Effective orifice area is plotted against frequency, according to the Gorlin formula

$$\frac{\text{AFlow}}{44.5 \ \sqrt{\text{PLV}-\text{PAO}}}$$

(AFlow = aortic valve flow; other values see Table 1).

♦ (SJM) shows the best values
○ (OS) and ✦ (HK) follow closely behind
■ (BSCC) falls off at low frequencies and improves at high frequencies
△ (BS) performs well at low frequencies and falls off at high frequencies

51

percent of stroke volume at four different stroke volumes and two different frequencies. The closing volumes of the St. Jude Medical valve amounted to 5.1 ± 1.3%, the Björk-Shiley Spherical valve followed with 5.8 ± 2.5%, the Björk-Shiley Convexo-Concave with 6.0 ± 1.3%, the Omniscience with 7.4 ± 0.9%, and the Medtronic Hall with 8.5 ± 1.7%.

Static and dynamic components of prosthetic valve performance

A pulse duplicator was developed because sufficient comparative in vitro data on valve performance are frequently not available for new mechanical valvular prostheses. In vivo studies do not usually separate valve performance into dynamic and static components. The first is dependent on the mechanical parts and the second on size, profile of the cage and the bulk of the suture ring in relation to the aortic diameter (1,6,7). Static components of valvular performance are relatively predictable, but dynamic components are subject to less predictable variations, depending on the alteration of pressure/flow/frequency relationships. Therefore, valves should always be tested under the dynamic conditions of a pulse duplicator.

Any artificial circulation will exhibit certain idiosyncrasies depending on the compliance of pulse duplicator compartments, the mode of fluid displacement and the type of liquid used for simulation. In this respect, glycerol/water mixtures are suboptimal, since they simulate the viscosity of blood, not its density. A pumping mechanism which uses gas for displacement of the stroke volume is optimal when high frequencies are required, but causes decreased accuracy of volume displacement measurement during changes of frequency.

In the present model, frequency and stroke volume were preselected by machine settings, and constant performance was observed over 10 minutes. Measurements were then taken over 3 minutes. Displacement volume was measured directly, and frequency was calculated from tracings taken during each recording period. The data presented in this paper are from six frequency settings and one displacement setting for each valve. Correlations of frequency and flow were nearly linear for all valves. The gradients were also nearly linear in relationship to frequency and reached nearly to 90 mm Hg at 120 bpm with corresponding flows of nearly 9000 ml/min. These absolute values are higher than expected from data obtained in vivo, when the same valves were tested at similar flow and frequency (17).

The causes of this phenomenon may be the use of 36% glycerol/water mixture, which can only simulate blood and produces higher gradients than water. In addition, the outflow track of our simulator is narrower, longer and stiffer than the left ventricular outflow track in the human heart and, therefore, may augment the stenosis of the valve. Moreover, peak gradients at maximum flow are reported rather than mean systolic gradients. In our view, it is sufficient to express the mechanical properties of valvular prostheses in gradient/stroke volume (mm Hg/ml) at a given frequency, since this term includes flow, frequency and pressure drop across the outflow track. We prefer this simple description of valvular function to more complicated expressions, such as loss of energy (5) or efficiency units (2), since these units require translation to the clinician who, in his daily routine, is restricted to pressure and flow data. The data obtained show clear separation of the Björk Shiley-Spherical and the St. Jude Medical bileaflet valves at frequencies greater than 80 bpm, which has to be interpreted as a consequence of the better hydrodynamic qualities of the St. Jude Medical valve.

The Gorlin formula (14) for calculation of effective orifice area has been commonly used to determine the necessity of aortic valve replacement. A number of authors have reported that this formula may not be equally applicable to artificial valves (15–17). The observed decrease of effective orifice area with frequency as obtained with this method does not necessarily represent the hydrodynamic performance of these valves. In the Gorlin formula, aortic valve flow is determined by systolic ejection time and cardiac output, divided by the square root of the gradient and multiplied by a constant. Both terms in the numerator decrease with frequency while the gradient increases, which results in a smaller effective orifice area.

Use of the Gorlin formula for this purpose may appear questionable, but effective orifice area remains one of the parameters frequently used to report the properties of artificial valves (2, 8). Disregarding the absolute values of these calculations, the use of Gorlin's formula appears acceptable for comparing valves under identical conditions, since it clearly separates the performance of the five valves tested at low and high frequencies.

Evaluation of prosthetic valve hemodynamics by in vitro tests

In summary, this study indicates that simulator studies are necessary to compare the hemodynamic properties of artificial valves. The results of such studies may be altered by the specific hydrodynamic or mechanical properties of the apparatus. The St. Jude Medical bileaflet valve in our pulse duplicator offered some hydrodynamic advantages over the Björk-Shiley Convexo-Concave, the Medtronic Hall and the Omniscience valves. The Björk-Shiley Spherical valve has to be considered less advantageous.

However, differences in hydraulic performance are of minor importance and more prominent differences in valvular performances after implantation are caused by the valvular profile and the suture ring, thus determining residual stenosis. These differences can probably be detected under clinical testing conditions, but need to be distinguished from the actual mechanical performance of a valve.

References

1. Snobank DS, Yoganathan AP, Meyer MS et al (1980) In vitro comparison of the performance indices of prosthetic aortic heart valves. AAMI 15:206 (Abstr)
2. Gabbay S, Yellin SL, Frishman WH et al (1980) In vitro hydrodynamic comparison of St. Jude, Björk-Shiley and Hall-Kaster valves. Trans Am Soc Artif Intern Organs 26:231
3. Emery RW, Palmquist WE, Mettler E et al (1978) A new cardiac valve prosthesis: In vitro results. Trans Am Soc Artif Intern Organs 24:550
4. Umezu M, Tomino T, Kawazoe K (1980) Mechanical simulator for the evaluation of hemodynamic performance of artificial heart valves. Proc 2nd Internat Conference of Mechanics in Medicine and Biology, Osaka: 136
5. Scotten LN, Racca RG, Nugent AH et al (1981) New tilting disc valve prostheses. J Thorac Cardiovasc Surg 82:136
6. Wright JTM (1972) Prosthetic heart valves: Clinical requirements, design and performance. Biomed Engineering 7:160
7. Köhler J, Ehrentraut G (1980) Druckverluste von Björk-Shiley CC und Omniscience Herzklappen im Modellkreislauf. Biomedizinische Technik 25: Suppl 73
8. Gombrich PP, Villafana MA, Palmquist WE (1979) From concept to clinical: The St. Jude Medical bileaflet pyrolytic carbon cardiac valve. AAMI Proc 14:1
9. Gottwik M, Neumair K, Tessari R et al (1982) Comparison of Björk-Shiley ABP and St. Jude Medical prostheses in a newly developed pulse duplicator. J Cardiovasc Surg 23:34
10. Tsakiris GA, Rastelli GAB, Banchero N et al (1966) Hemodynamic effects of implanting a rigid ring in the annulus of the mitral valve. Am J Cardiol 17:141

11. Kaster RL, Lillehei CW, Starek PJ (1970) The Lillehei-Kaster pivoting disc aortic prosthesis and a comparative study of its pulsatile flow characteristics with four other prostheses. Trans Am Soc Artif Intern Organs 16:233
12. Reif TM, Huffstutler MC (1979) A preliminary flow study of a two-dimensional model of a concave-convex pivoting disc prosthetic heart valve. Proc Seventh N Engl Bioeng Conf, p 209
13. Björk VO, Book K, Holmgren A (1973) Significance of position and opening angle of the Björk-Shiley tilting disc valve in mitral surgery. Scand J Thorac Cardiovasc Surg 7:187
14. Gorlin R, Gorlin SG (1951) Hydraulic formula for calculation of the area of the stenotic mitral valve, other cardiac valves, and central circulatory shunts. Am Heart J 41:1
15. Aaslid R, Levang O, Fröysaker T et al (1975) In situ elevation of the aortic pivoting disc valve prosthesis. Scand J Thorac Cardiovasc Surg 9:81
16. Köhler J, Baghai N (1982) Determination of the heart valve orifice. In: Bleifeld W, Harder D, Leetz HK et al (eds) Proceedings of the World Congress of Medical Physics and Biomedical Engineering. MPBE Publishing, Hamburg, p 5
17. Thormann J, Gottwik M, Schlepper M et al (1981) Hemodynamic alterations induced by isoproterenol and pacing after aortic valve replacement with the Björk-Shiley or St. Jude Medical prosthesis. Circulation 63:895

Authors' address:

Dr. Martin Gottwik
Kerckhoff-Klinik
Benekestrasse 4–6
D–6350 Bad Nauheim
F.R.G.

Is the Late Outcome of Heart Valve Replacement Influenced by the Hemodynamics of the Heart Valve Substitute?

D. Horstkotte, F. Loogen and W. Bircks

Although many of the problems of the early years of heart valve replacement seem to be solved, other problems still remain. For example, the high operative mortality of the early years has decreased to less than 5% (1); today operative long-term complications (2) and insufficient recovery from preoperative myocardial dysfunction (3) are of much more concern.

How to determine the late outcome of heart valve replacement

From the start, frequency of mechanical dysfunction, prosthetic valve endocarditis, thromboembolic and other complications, have been compared for the various valves. How hemodynamics of a prosthesis influences late clinical outcome has attracted little attention. This is because statements about the probability of complications of artificial heart valves can be made a few years after implantation and can easily be compared with results of other prostheses if patient groups are comparable and the same statistical methods are used (4). The consequences of a decrease in ventricular function and the patient's physical capacity can only be evaluated several years postoperatively; and even then the causal relationships are hard to prove because of the variety of influences on long-term outcome.

It has been shown that the life expectancy of patients with severe heart valve lesions has been remarkably increased, due to the improvement of perioperative and postoperative management (5); now it has become a matter of growing importance to determine if the late outcome of valvular patients is influenced by the hemodynamics of the implanted heart valve substitute.

Table 1. How to determine late outcome after valve replacement

---
- Subjective improvement
- Improvement of functional capacity
- Improvement of hemodynamics
- Cumulative survival rates
- Cumulative event-free rates

However, before this can be determined, one has to ascertain the parameters of the late outcome. The parameters listed in Table 1 are influenced by the flow characteristics of the chosen valve type. In an individual patient's case, however, it may be difficult to calculate how much the hemodynamics of a prosthetic device influence the outcome.

55

For these reasons one should determine how the objective data of hemodynamics and complication rates affect the subjective data of patient complaints.

Subjective improvement due to hemodynamic alterations after prosthetic valve replacement

The correlation of less individual complaints to postoperative hemodynamic normalization, especially the pressures in pulmonary circulation, seems obvious. The correlation of the patient's complaints about shortness of breath, and the pressures in pulmonary circulation verified by floating catheter studies at rest and under ergometric exercise, is good when mean data are considered.

The correlation of subjective postoperative improvement with changes of mean pulmonary artery pressure has also, in our experience, resulted in a very good correspondence. We have used the very strict categories of the New York Heart Association (NYHA) (7) (Figure 1). Patients who could not be classified into a better NYHA category showing postoperative improvement, had an identical or only slightly decreased mean pulmonary artery pressure (PAP) after mitral valve replacement. In the majority of these patients, PAP was pathological at rest and already increasing markedly even under light bicycle exercise. Patients who improved one or two NYHA Classes showed an average decrease of PAP to normal values. In particular, patients with an improvement of one NYHA Classification had

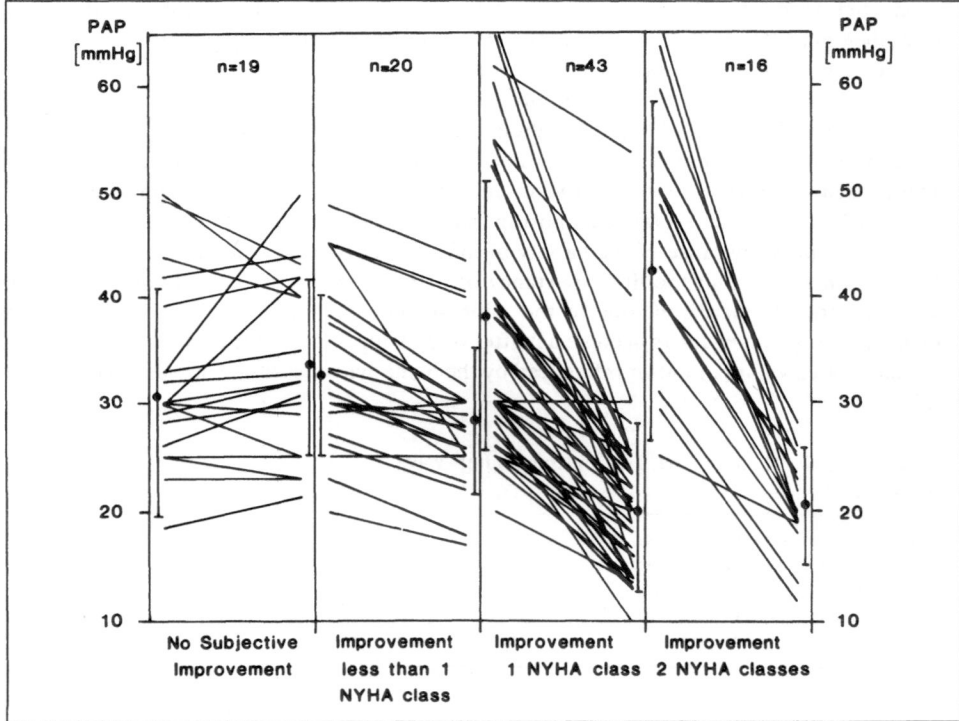

Fig. 1. Correlation between clinical improvement according to the New York Heart Association's Classification of clinical severity of valvular heart lesions (NYHA) and mean pulmonary artery pressures (PAP) before and after mitral valve replacement in 98 patients with randomized mitral valve replacement with Björk-Shiley, Lillehei-Kaster, and Starr-Edwards prostheses.

nonphysiological PAP increase under bicycle exercise, while most of the patients with an improvement of two NYHA Classes showed normal PAP values up to an exercise capacity of 75 watts.

After mitral valve replacement, a correlation between increased PAP and transprosthetic gradient is only justified if a normal left ventricular function is present and the PVR is not increased. Even with an increased preoperative pulmonary vascular resistance (PVR) following mitral valve replacement for mitral stenosis or combined mitral valve lesions, there is mostly a decrease of resistance in the pulmonary circulation. This decrease, in relation to the duration of the disease, does not always reach normal values (8).

This positive postoperative correlation of symptoms and hemodynamics is found in contrast to other studies, which report a low correlation of preoperative symptoms, functional capacity and exercise hemodynamics in patients with heart valve diseases (9).

Irreversible myocardial damage before valve replacement may postoperatively cause increased pulmonary artery pressures. To exclude persistent left ventricular dysfunction and to make clinical and hemodynamic results of different prostheses comparable with the prospective randomized implantation (10), an exact determination of left ventricular end-diastolic pressure (LVEDP), PVR and transmitral gradients is indispensable. By doing this,

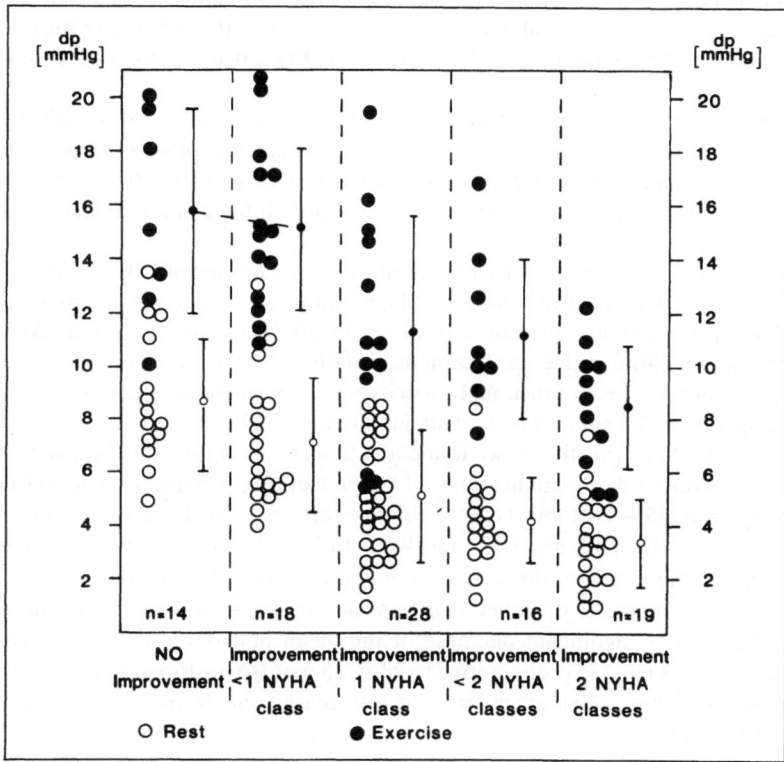

Fig. 2. Correlation between clinical improvement according to the New York Heart Association's Classification (NYHA) and the transmitral gradients (dp) after randomized mitral valve replacement with Bjrök-Shiley, Lillehei-Kaster and Starr-Edwards prostheses in 95 patients measured by transseptal and retrograde catheterization. The open circles represent the measurements at rest, the closed circles under 30 watts bicycle exercise in the supine position.

left ventricular dysfunctions, increases of pulmonary resistance and other factors influencing pulmonary artery pressure can be excluded from the comparison, and the pressures measured in pulmonary circulation under rest and exercise conditions can be regarded as a direct consequence of disturbances of the blood flow through the prosthesis.

Figure 2 summarizes the correspondence between postoperative clinical improvement and transprosthetic pressure gradient measured at rest and under exercise by retrograde and transseptal catherization one year after randomized mitral valve replacement. Because none of these patients showed an increase of pulmonary vascular resistance of more than 300 $dyn \cdot sec \cdot cm^{-5}$ or a LVEDP increase of more than 12 mm Hg, a correlation between improved functional capacity or a decreased mean pulmonary artery pressure and the obstruction of blood flow through the artificial valve seems to be legitimate.

Improvement of functional capacity and postoperative central hemodynamics

The improvement experienced by patients after prosthetic valve replacement can be objectively compared with functional capacity before and after the operation. This can be done using a bicycle ergometer, a climbing step or a stair test. We use the stair test or a bicycle ergometer, because these examinations are easy to perform, and bicycle ergometry and climbing stairs are physical work (about 25%), nearly reaching the optimum efficiency of an isolated muscle (30%). With step climbing, however, the efficiency amounts to only about 19% (11).

During the stair test, patients climb at a constant speed of one step per second until they have to stop because of dyspnoea or muscular exhaustion. In this and other exercise tests, individual parameters, such as patient training conditions, also become effective. Comparisons of different patient groups are thus only valid if possible influencing parameters are randomized.

After valve replacement for a combined rheumatic mitral valve lesion with Björk-Shiley,[R] St. Jude Medical[R], Carpentier-Edwards[R], Ionescu-Shiley[R] and Hancock[R] valve prostheses, a mean functional improvement in the stair test of 40 to 100% can be expected. After prospective randomized mitral valve replacement, relative to the type of prostheses implanted, significant differences in functional capacity were documented in patient groups with identical preoperative clinical and hemodynamic findings (10).

In patients with a Björk-Shiley prosthesis, we found a 92% increase in functional capacity in the stair test. This corresponds to publications of other working groups, who found an increase in capacity from 35% to about 60% of the age-related normal value after mitral valve replacement (12). In patients who received Lillehei-Kaster prostheses under randomized conditions, the increase, however, amounted to only 45% (Figure 3).

The significantly higher increase of functional capacity in patients with Björk-Shiley prostheses also correlates to significant decrease of the mean pulmonary artery pressure (PAP) at rest from 35 ± 13 mm Hg preoperative to 23 ± 13 mm Hg postoperative, whereas the PAP in patients with Lillehei-Kaster[R] mitral valves decreased only from 35 ± 12 mm Hg to 30 ± 10 mm Hg (Figure 3).

The comparison of functional capacity under bicycle ergometer exercise in the supine position and the PAP of patients with Björk-Shiley and St. Jude Medical prostheses is documented in Figure 4. In the Björk-Shiley group the mean PAP was increased from 23 ± 8 mm Hg at rest, 36 ± 10 mm Hg at 30 W, 43 ± 10 mm Hg (60 W), 48 ± 11 mm Hg (90 W), 53 ± 16 mm Hg (120 W) up to 57 ± 16 mm Hg at a work load of 150 W. In the group

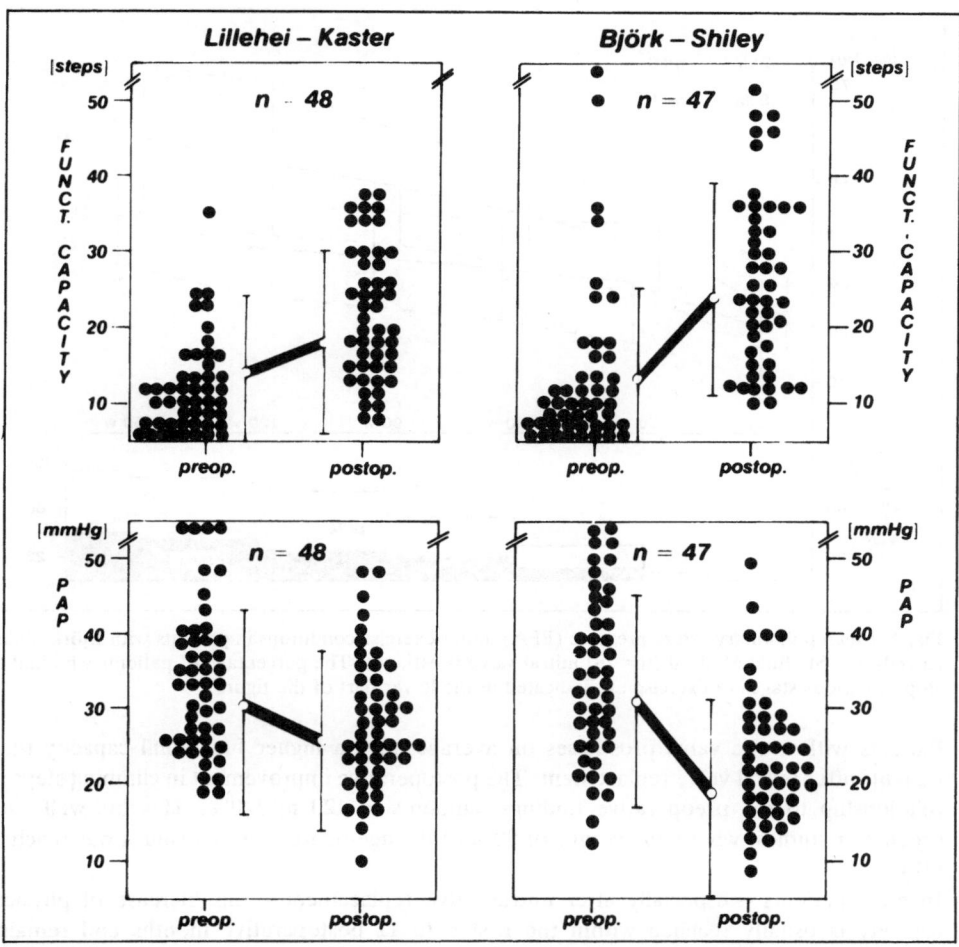

Fig. 3. Correlation between the functional capacity of patients after randomized Björk-Shiley and Lillehei-Kaster mitral valve replacement and the mean pulmonary artery pressure (PAP) pre- and postoperatively. Functional capacity was evaluated by a stair climbing test.

with the St. Jude Medical prostheses the PAP at rest (20 ± 10 mm Hg) and under all exercise conditions 29 ± 12 mm Hg (30 W); 32 ± 10 mm Hg (60 W); 35 ± 9 mm Hg (90 W); 36 ± 9 mm Hg (120 W); 43 ± 10 mm Hg (150 W) was lower than in the patient collective with Björk-Shiley mitral prostheses.

Corresponding to this higher PAP, the average patient with Björk-Shiley mitral prostheses finishes exercise under lower work loads. Thus, in the Björk-Shiley group only 71% of the patients reach a 60 W work load and only 29% reach a 120 W work load. However, in the St. Jude Medical collective, 89% reach 60 W work load and 74% reach 120 W work loads. The maximum work load of 150 W was reached by 49% of the patients with St. Jude Medical valves, and by only 11% of the patients with Björk-Shiley prostheses (Figure 4).

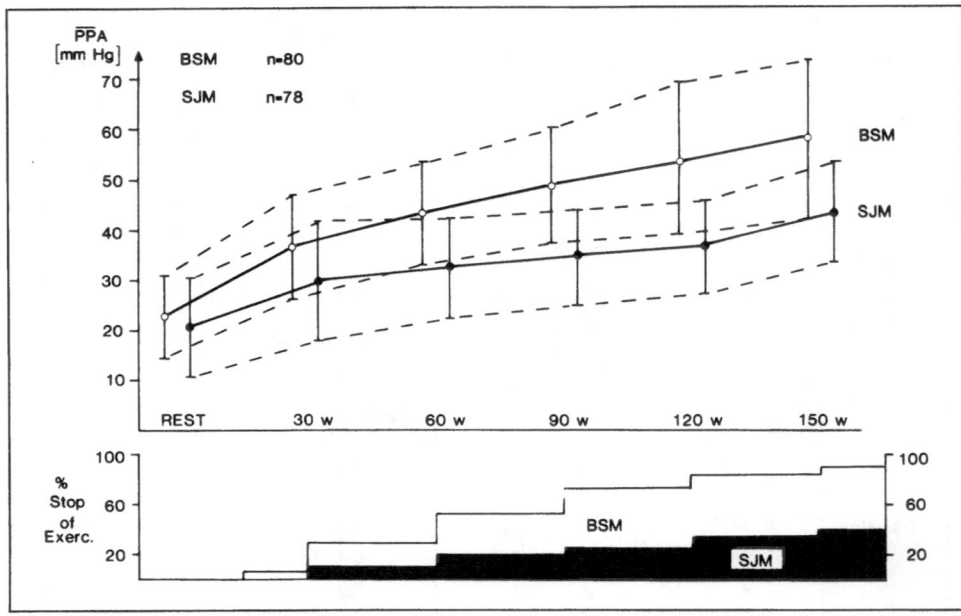

Fig. 4. Mean pulmonary artery pressure (PPA) under exercise conditions in patients with Björk-Shiley (n=80) and St. Jude Medical (n= 78) mitral valve prostheses. The percentage of patients who had to stop at various stages of exercise are indicated in the lower part of the figure.

Patients with aortic valve prostheses on average have a higher functional capacity than patients after mitral valve replacement. The postoperative improvement in climbing steps in relationship to the preoperative findings, amounts to 120 to 140%. This fits well with ergometer studies, where an average of 80% of the age-related normal values was reached (12).

In most patients – especially after mitral valve replacement – this increase of physical capacity is usually reached within the first 6 to 12 postoperative months and remains constant during follow-up, as long as no prosthetic malfunction or myocardial dysfunction occurs. The low increase of physical capacity after mitral valve replacements, as compared to that of patients with aortic valve prostheses, can be explained by hemodynamic disturbances with persistent postoperative atrial fibrillation. In relation to the duration of the arrhythmia existing, the conversion of atrial fibrillation after mitral valve replacement is successful in only a small percentage of patients. On the other hand, it is caused by the increase of diastolic pressure gradients across the mitral prostheses as the heart rate increases under exercise.

Figure 5 illustrates this exponential increase of the transmitral pressure gradients with the decrease of the diastolic left ventricular filling time concomitant with the increase of heart rate, for example under physical exercise.

At a stroke volume of 50 mL and a diastolic filling time (T_D) of 500 msec the quotient of pressure gradient and stroke volume (dp/SV) amounts to 0.056 mm Hg $\times$ mL^{-1}. At this stroke volume the patient will have a transmitral gradient of 2.8 mm Hg. This corresponds to a hemodynamically noneffective mitral stenosis. At the same stroke volume and with an increase in heart rate, therefore a decrease of the diastolic filling time to 200 msec, the

60

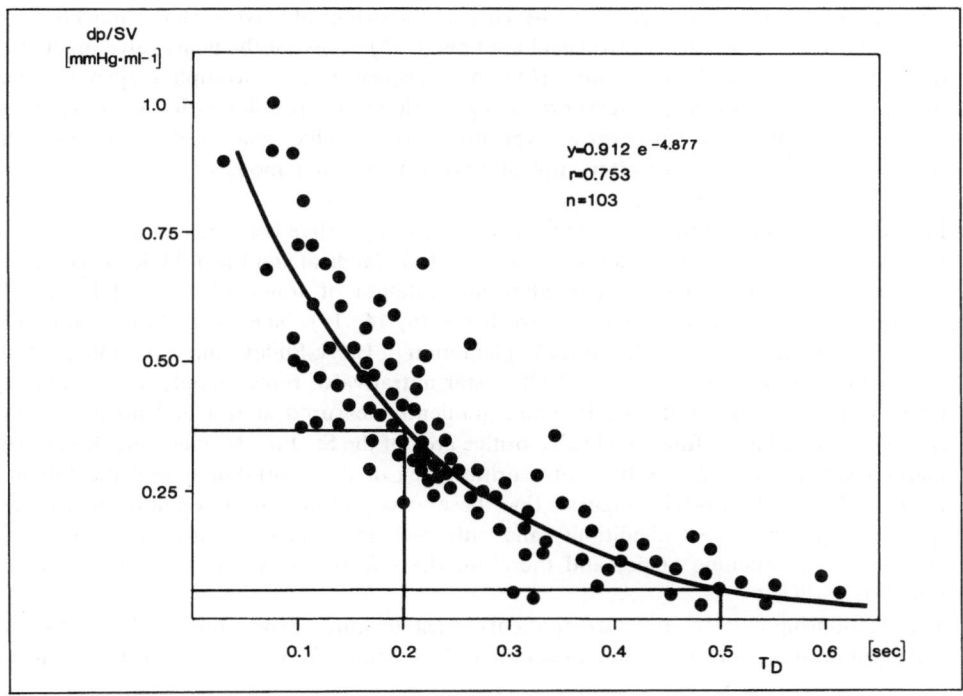

Fig. 5. Pressure gradient per ml stroke volume (dp/SV) versus diastolic filling time (T$_D$) in different mitral valve prostheses. Indicated are the values of dp/SV for a diastolic filling time of 0.5 and 0.2 sec.

quotient dp/SV increases to 0.36 mm Hg × mL^{-1}. This is equivalent to a transmitral pressure gradient of 18 mm Hg and therefore to a severe mitral stenosis.

From these data it is clear that most of the patients have inadequate relief of mitral valve obstruction under exercise. Functional capacity remains more or less significantly reduced after mitral valve replacement. The percentage of patients with mitral valve implants who return to work postoperatively is lower than in the group with isolated aortic valve replacement (14).

Postoperative improvement of central hemodynamics and flow/pressure relationships of prosthetic heart valves

If there are no differences in mean LVEDP or PVR and the complaints lessen and the functional capacity increases, showing a close correlation to decrease of mean pulmonary artery pressure (PAP) after randomized mitral valve replacement, the different pressures in the pulmonary circulation are direct consequences of high transprosthetic gradients.

All artificial valves produce a pronounced obstruction to forward blood flow corresponding to individual technical parameters. The space required for the sewing ring and valve housing affect higher transprosthetic pressure gradients the more the valve orifice area is narrowed. The more unfavorable the ratio of effective to total valve orifice area is, the more unfavorable are the hemodynamic properties of the given prosthesis (14).

The ratio of effective prosthetic orifice area to total orifice area after excision of the native valve, however, is not only determined by the relationship between the outer and inner diameter of the artificial valve, but especially by the extent of valve occluder movement in the bloodstream which also obstructs blood flow (6,15). Some of the heart valve prostheses developed show poor clinical results (16) as a consequence of an incomplete opening of the tilting disc, in spite of in vitro tests predicting excellent flow profiles with low pressure loss across the prosthesis. Even improved versions of these valves could not always solve the problems, so clinical results after implantation of these later models fall behind those of other mechanical valves (17).

For those mitral valve prostheses we studied, the postoperative hemodynamic improvement expressed in decrease of PAP and LAP after St. Jude Medical and Björk-Shiley mitral valve replacement is more marked than after implantation of Ionescu-Shiley, Hall-Kaster[R], Lillehei-Kaster and Starr-Edwards[R] prostheses (6, 14, 18). The lower flow disturbance found in pulse duplicator studies after implantation of Björk-Shiley, and especially St. Jude Medical prostheses, (and not after Hall-Kaster mitral valve replacement), corresponds to lower transprosthetic gradients. Pressure gradients measured at rest and under exercise correspond to a higher functional valve orifice area of the St. Jude Medical prostheses. The marked increase of the effective valve orifice area of the Björk-Shiley and the Lillehei-Kaster valves under exercise suggests that these valves do not always open to their design specifications under rest conditions, and only with increasing pressure gradients under exercise is the opening angle, and therefore the effective valve orifice area, increased (16, 18).

The relationship between pressure gradients, diastolic mitral flows and calculated effective valve orifice areas at rest and under exercise is documented for 6 types of prostheses studied

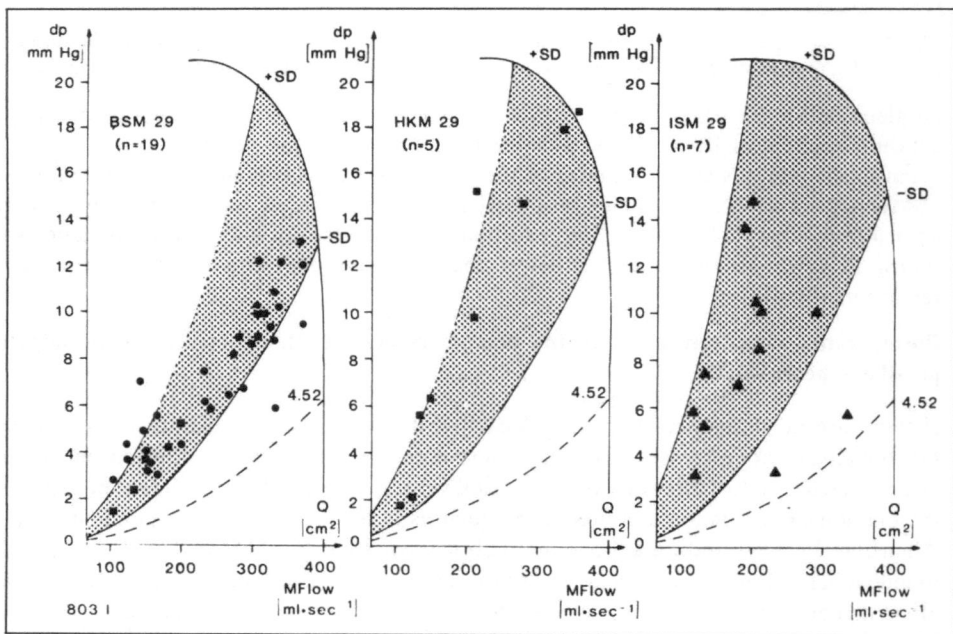

Fig. 6. Pressure-flow relationship for Björk-Shiley, Hall-Kaster and Ionescu-Shiley mitral valve prostheses of 29-mm external diameter. dp = transmitral gradient measured by transseptal and retrograde catheterization; MFlow = diastolic mitral flow per second. The geometric orifice area (Q) is marked with dashed lines. The area between the standard deviations is shaded.

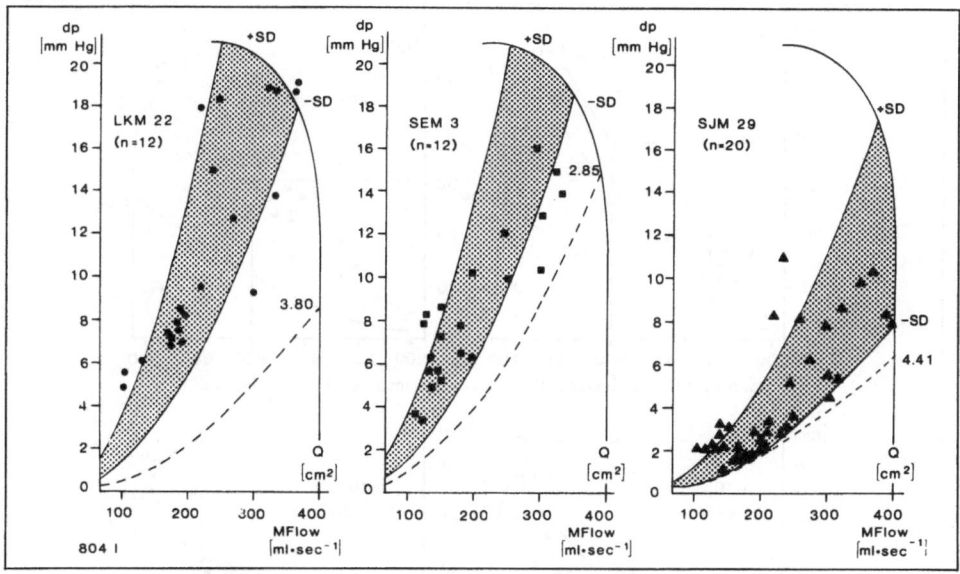

Fig. 7. Relationship between pressure gradient (dp), diastolic mitral flow (MFlow), and geometric valve orifice area (Q) in Lillehei-Kaster, Starr-Edward, and St. Jude Medical mitral valve prostheses with identical external valve diameters of 29 mm.

in Figures 6 and 7. The geometric orifice area for the mitral prostheses of almost equivalent size (29 mm outer diameter) is smaller for the Starr-Edwards and the Lillehei-Kaster prostheses than for the other valve types (18). The difference between geometric and effective valve orifice area is very marked for all mitral valves in the Hall-Kaster and Lillehei-Kaster group and is inhomogeneous for the Ionescu-Shiley prostheses. After Björk-Shiley, Starr-Edwards and St. Jude Medical mitral valve replacement, this difference is less extensive. This implicates lower transprosthetic pressure gradients after Björk-Shiley and especially after St. Jude Medical implantations when comparing mitral valve prostheses of equivalent outer diameter under identical mitral flows. Similar results are found in the comparison of Björk-Shiley and St. Jude Medical aortic valve prostheses of the same outer diameter under rest and exercise conditions (15).

The geometric orifice area of the 25 mm Björk-Shiley prostheses is 3.1 cm². At rest, this geometric orifice area is by no means attained in our measurements, so that the mean effective valve orifice area in the 16 patients shown in Figure 8 is 1.8 cm². The average pressure gradient at rest and at a mean systolic flow of 320 mL/sec is calculated to be 16 mm Hg.

After 3 minutes of 30 W bicycle exercise, the average transprosthetic gradient is 24 mm Hg. The effective valve orifice area is higher than that under rest conditions. Under 60 W the average gradient increases up to 26 mm Hg and the effective valve orifice area is 2.2 cm². At 90 W the effective valve orifice area is 2.3 cm² and the mean pressure gradient is 29 mm Hg (Figure 8). However, for the 25 mm St. Jude Medical aortic valve prostheses a significant difference between effective and geometric valve orifice area (Figure 9) was not found in comparison with the equally sized Björk-Shiley valves; the systolic pressure gradients are significantly lower.

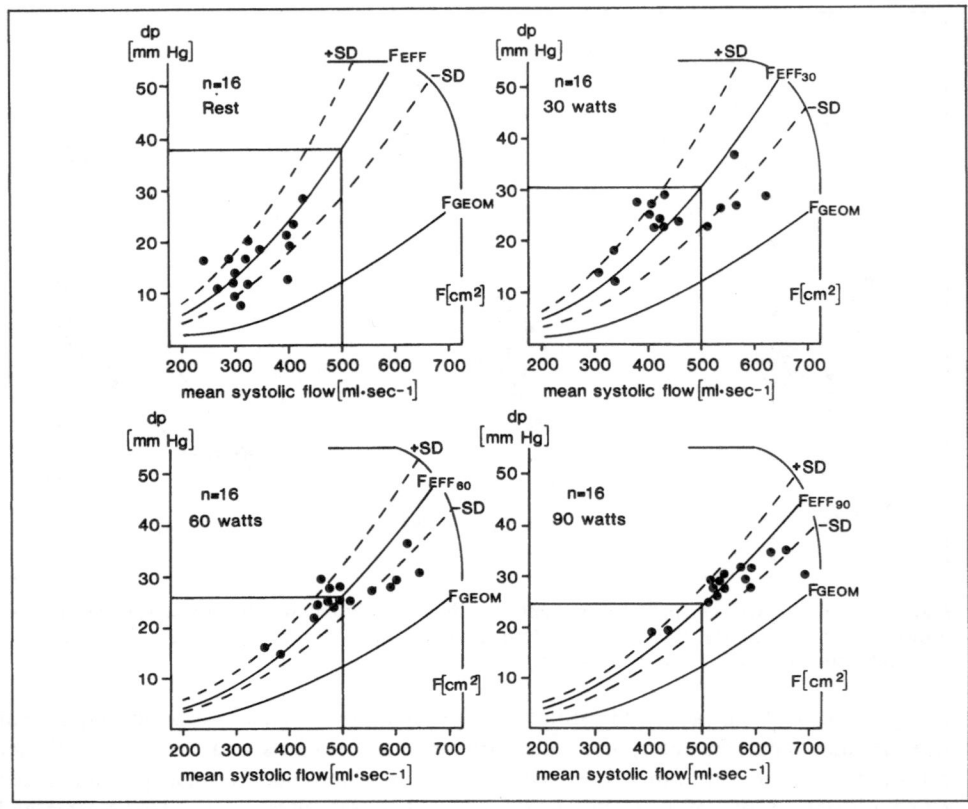

Fig. 8. Flow/pressure relationship in Björk-Shiley 25-mm aortic prostheses at rest and during exercise of 30, 60 and and 90 watts.

These data elucidate the fact that differences between geometric and effective valve orifice areas are not a systematic error of measurement, although it is obvious that the Gorlin formula has important limitations in calculating orifice areas of prosthetic valves reliably (19). However, using the same formula in calculating the orifice area for the St. Jude Medical valves, the differences between calculated and geometric orifice area are small.

Influence of prosthetic valve hemodynamics on the restoration of left ventricular impairment

Besides the restitution of valve function, the extent of normalization of a disturbed left ventricular function distinctly influences the postoperative result. This left ventricular impairment is probably related to the compromised left ventricular inotropic state prior to surgery or to intraoperative myocardial damage. Also, the residual obstruction to forward blood flow caused by the prosthetic valve itself may be responsible.

To test the influence of residual transprosthetic gradients on the normalization of the function of the left ventricle, we studied the postoperative results in 33 patients with considerable left ventricular dysfunction preoperatively, in relation to the type of prosthesis implanted.

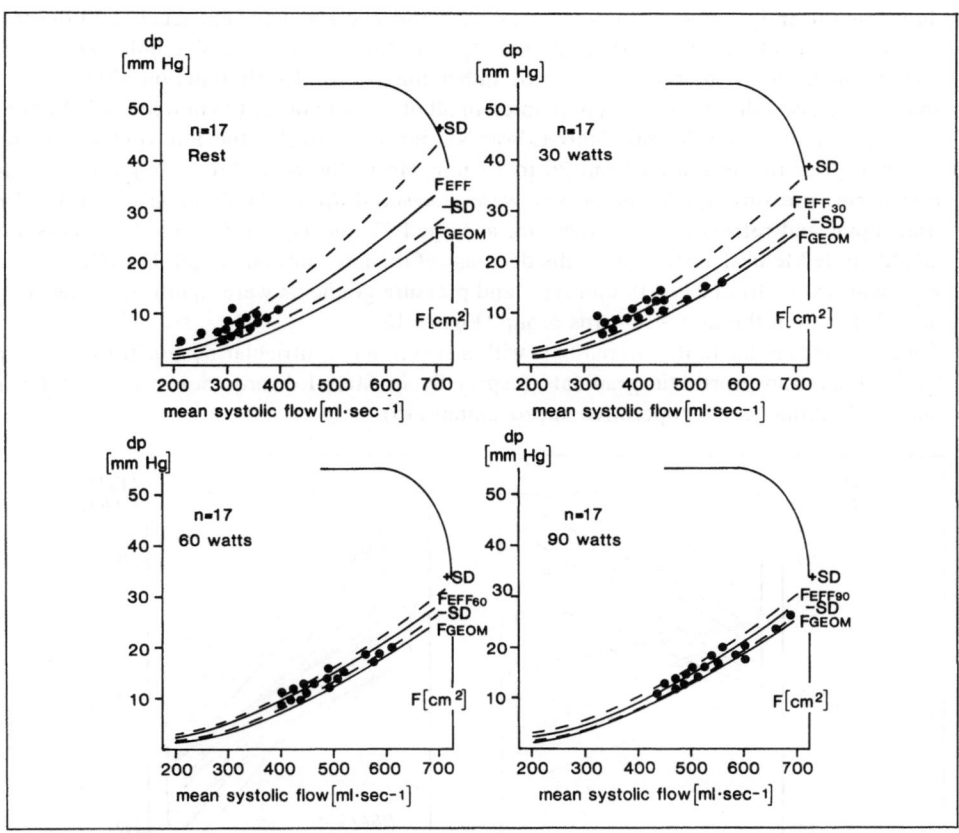

Fig. 9. Flow/pressure relationship in St. Jude Medical 25-mm aortic valve prostheses at rest and during exercise of 30, 60 and 90 watts.

Table 2. Aortic valve replacement for aortic stenosis (severe LV-dysfunction).

PREOP.	A(n=16) SE-ball valves	B(n=17) BS or SJ-valves
LVEDP	26.1 ± 5.2 mm Hg	27.2 ± 4.2 mm Hg
EF	$29.8 \pm 5.5\%$	$28.6 \pm 5.4\%$
CI	$1.84 \pm 0.32 \, 1 \cdot m^{-2}$	$1.67 \pm 0.43 \, 1 \cdot m^{-2}$
SVJ	19.5 ± 5.1 ml $\cdot m^{-2}$	19.4 ± 5.7 ml $\cdot m^{-2}$

Group A consists of 16 patients in whom a Starr-Edwards ball valve was implanted; group B consists of 17 patients who received Björk-Shiley or St. Jude Medical prostheses some years later.

In Table 2, 16 patients who received Starr-Edwards prostheses between 1972 and 1977 are summarized as Group A. Group B consists of 17 patients with either Björk-Shiley or St. Jude Medical valves implanted between 1974 and 1980. Most of these patients had been operated on during the same time interval and virtually the same operative and myocardial preservation techniques had been used. The preoperative hemodynamic status does not differ significantly between these two groups; the average left ventricular end-diastolic pressure gradient was higher than 25 mm Hg. Ejection fraction, cardiac index and stroke volume index were markedly reduced, indicating severe LV-dysfunction (Table 2). A similar-sized prosthesis had been implanted in all of these patients (23 mm St. Jude Medical and Björk-Shiley and 24 mm Starr-Edwards). Postoperatively, the left ventricular end-diastolic pressure decreased from 26 to 22 mm Hg in the Starr-Edwards group and the transaortic pressure gradients, which were measured from simultaneous records after transseptal and retrograde catherization, averaged 27 mm Hg. In Group B, Björk-Shiley and St. Jude Medical aortic valves, the decrease of the left ventricular end-diastolic pressure was significant – from 27 to 15 mm Hg – and pressure gradients were significantly lower (17 mm Hg) than in the Starr-Edwards group (Figure 10).

These findings indicate that in patients with a severe left ventricular dysfunction preoperatively, high transprosthetic gradients (especially in Starr-Edwards aortic implants) may negatively influence postoperative improvement (15).

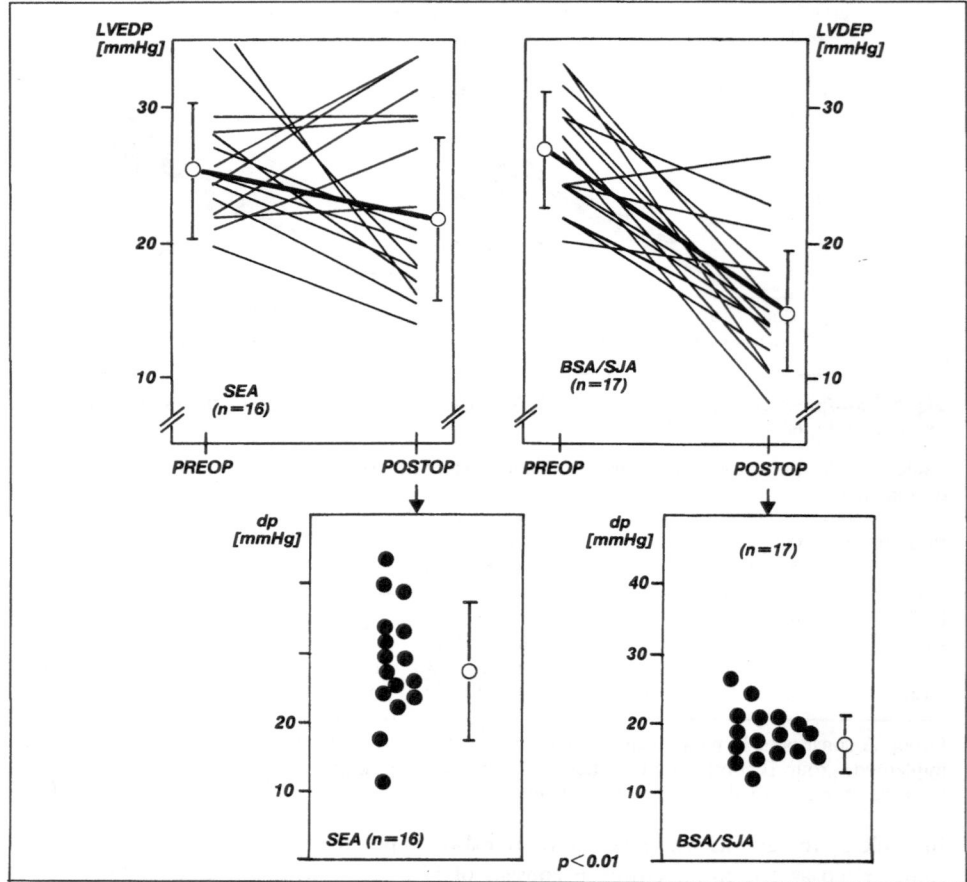

Fig. 10. Left ventricular end-diastolic pressure (LVEDP) before and after Starr-Edwards (SEA) and St. Jude Medical or Björk-Shiley aortic valve replacement (BSA/SJA) versus the postoperative transaortic gradients in both groups.

Influence of postoperative hemodynamics on complication rates

Prosthetic valve-related or valve-induced complications limit overall success of valve replacement. The incidence of these complications, in relationship to the types of prostheses implanted, has been documented. However, little attention has been paid to the influence of hemodynamic properties of the prostheses on these complications.

Complications after prosthetic heart valve implantation are influenced by 5 factors: therapeutic factors, extracardial factors, prosthetic valve material, cardiac factors and prosthetic valve hemodynamics (Table 3).

Table 3. Factors influencing complications after heart valve replacement.

Therapeutic factors	Extracardial factors	Prosthetic valve material	Cardiac factors	Prosthetic valve hemodynamics
Hemorrhage				
Prosthetic valve endocarditis				
Thrombembolic complications				
	Tissue ingrowth			
		Mechanical dysfunction		
		Periprosthetic leaks		
				Hemolysis

Mechanical dysfunction of mechanical valves (20) and xenografts are normally consequences of defects of the prosthetic material. Paraprosthetic leaks (21) can be the result of insufficient sewing rings or severe calcification, unstable sutures, and florid, infectious endocarditis. Hindered movement of the valve occluder by tissue ingrowth is usually caused by extracardial factors; however, sometimes it can be caused by the material of the sewing ring and the design of the artificial valve. Prosthetic valve endocarditis (22) occurring later that 2 months postoperatively and not directly attributed to the operation, usually appears for extracardial reasons and without effective prophylaxis. The tissue of xenografts more frequently causes inflammation while patients with mechanical prostheses may have a more severe course of infection. Hemorrhages are very distinctly related to anticoagulant treatment (23). Interactions of anticoagulants and variant medical or nutritive factors are well known.

Hemolysis and thromboembolic complications are influenced by the prosthetic hemodynamics. Chronic intravascular hemolysis has its origin in mechanical damage of red blood cells. The cause of this erythrocyte damage is shearing stress on the formed blood elements and is the consequence of streaming turbulences or high flow velocity, pressure losses at the prosthesis and damage occurring when the valve occluder hits the valve ring (24, 25). High velocities are expected with forward flow through the narrowed valve diameter or leakage through the not completely closed prosthesis. The change in flow profile with increased pressure gradients at the artificial heart valve results from higher turbulences. The traumatization of the formed blood elements caused by this mechanism can also lead to the liberation of thrombocyte-specific enzymes and can initiate the formation of platelet aggregates. Thromboembolic events generated by formation of thrombi close to the prosthesis are partially due to the hemodynamics disturbed by the prosthesis. Additionally, and probably to a high degree, the thrombogenicity of the prosthetic material, other cardiac factors such as size of the left atrium and the left ventricle, ventricle function and arrhythmias play an important role (26). Also the extracardiac factors which with today's examination methods cannot yet be sufficiently documented such as coagulability, are of importance (Table 3).

The close correlation between hemodynamic parameters that indicate shear stresses in turbulent and rapid blood flow, and the degree of intravascular hemolysis, is today sufficiently documented (24). Besides this red cell traumatization, other formed blood elements are also damaged. The damage to thrombocytes results in the liberation of thrombocyte-specific enzymes such as ß-thromboglobulin and platelet factor 4 which are of special importance for clot formation (28). Therefore it seems obvious that there is also a correlation between the hemodynamic properties of prosthetic heart valves and the

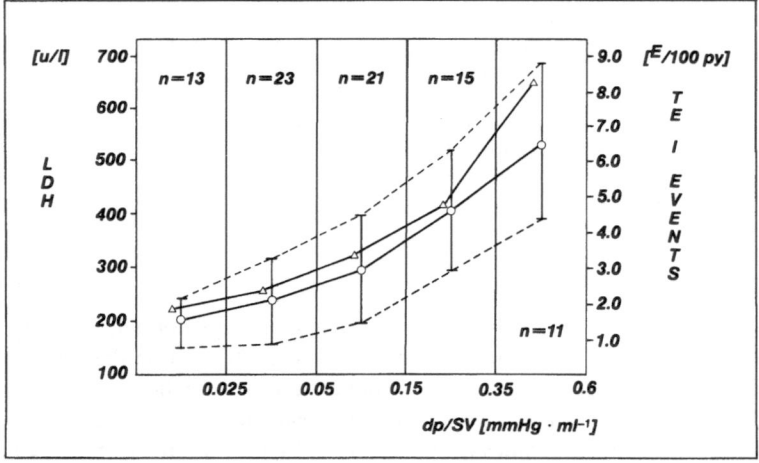

Fig. 11. Degree of hemolysis as indicated by the LDH-levels (−O−) and incidence of thromboembolic events (TE-events) expressed as TE-events per 100 patient-years (py) (−△−) versus pressure gradients per ml stroke volume (dp/SV).

68

incidence of thromboembolic complications (29). Investigations into these relationships are still at an early stage. Controlled or randomized studies are not yet available.

For 83 patients extensively studied in our clinic with right heart, transseptal and retrograde catherization at rest and under exercise, however, a close correlation between the pressure/ flow relationship of the artificial valves, the degree of intravascular hemolysis and the incidence of thromboembolic events could be documented. Figure 11 illustrates that in the group with 13 patients, where the quotient of pressure gradient (dp) and stroke volume (SV) was lower than 0.025 mm Hg $\cdot$ mL^{-1}, the hemolysis measured by the prototypic hemolysis parameter LDH was a mean of 200 U/L. The incidence of thromboembolism in this group was below 2.0 events per 100 patient-years. Of the 21 patients with a quotient dp/SV of 0.05 to 0.15 mm Hg $\cdot$ mL^{-1}, however, we found a mean LDH of 280 U/L and an incidence of thromboembolism of 3.5 events per 100 patient-years. For patients with very high pressure gradients and a quotient dp/SV of more than 0.35 mm Hg $\cdot$ mL^{-1} the mean LDH was 500 U/L. The risk of thromboembolism in this group was 8 events per 100 patient-years. None of these patients had a malfunction of the prosthesis.

Hemodynamic influence on late outcome after heart valve replacement

The results presented above have been composed of consecutive and randomized operative series and follow-up groups. Therefore, they cannot stand against the strict criteria of controlled clinical studies. Controlled clinical studies cannot be performed by only one center because of the low event incidence of such complications and the high requirements of complex hemodynamic studies with consecutive patient groups.

In spite of this, the data show that the hemodynamic properties of the artificial valve influence the subjective result, the functional result and the normalization of the central hemodynamics. The influence of the prosthetic hemodynamics on hemolysis is virtually unquestioned; the influence on thromboembolic, and perhaps some other complications, has scarcely been studied. However, correlations also appear likely for these factors.

Prosthetic hemodynamics is a decisive parameter in many respects for the late outcome after heart valve replacement.

References

1. Rodewald GM, Polonius MJ (1984) Cardiac surgery in the Federal Republic of Germany during 1983. A report by the German Society for Thoracic and Cardiovascular Surgery. Thorac Cardiovasc Surg 32: 395
2. Horstkotte D, Körfer R, Seipel L et al (1983) Late complications in patients with Björk-Shiley and St. Jude Medical heart valve replacement. Circulation 68 (Suppl II): 175
3. Mehmel HC, Hasper B, Zebe H et al (1978) Die linksventrikuläre Funktion bei Aortenklappen-stenose und -insuffizienz präoperativ und nach prothetischem Herzklappenersatz. Z Kardiol 67: 242
4. MacManus Q, Grunkemeier GL, Lambert LE al (1980) Year of operation as a risk factor in the late results of valve replacement. J Thorac Cardiovasc Surg 80: 834
5. Horstkotte D, Haerten, K, Krian A (1983) Der prothetische Herzklappenersatz: Natürlicher Verlauf operationswürdiger Herzklappenfehler. Möglichkeiten und klinische Ergebnisse der operativen Behandlung. Int Welt 6: 137
6. Horstkotte D, Haerten K, Seipel L et al (1983) Central hemodynamics at rest and during exercise after mitral valve replacement with different prostheses. Circulation 68 (Suppl II): 161
7. New York Heart Association (1964) The Criteria Committee of the New York Heart Association: Disease of the heart and blood vessels (nomenclature and criteria for diagnosis). Little Brown, Boston

8. Haerten K (1981) Möglichkeiten und Grenzen des prothetischen Herzklappenersatzes. Enke, Stuttgart, p 32
9. Kraus F, Rudolph W (1984) Symptoms, exercise capacity and exercise hemodynamics: Interrelationship and their role in quantification of valvular lesions. Herz 9: 187
10. Horstkotte D, Haerten K, Herzer JA et al (1983) Five-year results after randomized mitral valve replacement with Björk-Shiley, Lillehei-Kaster, and Starr-Edwards prostheses. Thorac Cardiovasc Surg 31: 206
11. Nowacki PE (1975) Der Wirkungsgrad bei ergometrischer Leistung. In: Mellerowicz H, Jokl E, Hansen G (eds) Ergebnisse der Ergometrie. Perimed, Erlangen, p 73
12. Carstens V, Behrenbeck DW, Higer HH (1983) Exercise capacity before and after cardiac valve surgery. Cardiology 70: 41
13. Führe U, Both A, Fischer G et al (1977) Evaluation of social status and hemodynamic results four to six years after prosthetic valve replacement. Z Kardiol 66: 251
14. Horstkotte D, Schulte HD, Körfer R et al (1982) Mitral valve replacement using different prosthetic valves. Int J Artif Organs 5: 177
15. Horstkotte D, Haerten K, Körfer R et al (1983) Hemodynamic findings at rest and during exercise after implantation of different aortic valve prostheses. Z Kardiol 72: 429
16. Sigwart U, Schmidt H, Gleichmann U et al (1976) In-vivo evaluation of the Lillehei-Kaster heart valve prosthesis. Ann Thorac Surg 22: 213
17. Ohlmeier, H, Mannebach H, Greitemeier A (1982) Clinical follow-up of patients after valve replacement with Omniscience cardiac valves: Can this valve be recommended? Z Kardiol 71: 350
18. Horstkotte D, Haerten K, Schulte HD et al (1983) Hemodynamic findings at rest and during exercise after implantation of different mitral valve prostheses with equal tissue annulus diameter. Z Kardiol 72: 385
19. Huhmann W, Köhler J Opening areas of arteficial valves. Z Kardiol 67: 672
20. Roberts WC (1976) Choosing a substitute cardiac valve. Type, size, surgeon. Am J Cardiol 38: 633
21. Burch GE, Giles TD (1974) Clinical evaluation of aortic and mitral valve prostheses. Am Heart J 92: 245
22. Horstkotte D, Körfer R, Loogen F et al (1984) Prosthetic valve endocarditis: Clinical findings and management. Eur Heart J 5 (Suppl C): 117
23. Horstkotte D, Körfer R, Budde Th et al (1983) Late complications following Björk-Shiley and St. Jude Medical heart valve replacement. Z Kardiol 72: 251
24. Horstkotte D, Haerten K, Leuner Ch et al (1978) Chronic intravascular hemolysis following mitral valve replacement with Björk-Shiley, Lillehei-Kaster, and Starr-Edwards prostheses. Z Kardiol 67: 629
25. Horstkotte D, Aul C, Seipel L et al (1983) Influence of valve type and valve functoin on chronic intravascular hemolysis following mitral and aortic valve replacement using alloprostheses. Z Kardiol 72: 119
26. Akutsu T, Modi VJ (1982) Fluid dynamics of several mechanical prosthetic heart valves using laser Doppler anemometer. Life Supp Syst, Proceedings IX Meeting ESAO: 102
27. Gentle CR (1982) Characterisation of leakage flow in cardiac valve prostheses. Life Supp Syst, Proceedings IX. Ann Meeting ESAO: 102
28. Heilmann E, Ritzenhöfer A, Achatzky et al (1978) Haptoglobin und Transferin nach künstlichem Herzklappenersatz. Herz/Kreisl 10: 84
29. Szekely P (1964) Systemic embolism and anticoagulant prophylaxis in rheumatic heart disease. Br Heart J 1964/I: 1209

Authors' address:
Dr. Dieter Horstkotte
Medizinische Klinik der
Universität Düsseldorf
Moorenstraße 5
D–4000 Düsseldorf
F.R.G.

When are Hemodynamics Important for the Selection of a Prosthetic Heart Valve?

G. Champsaur, M. Gressier, J. Ninet, J. P. Frieh, M. Elkirat,
P. Brule, A. Lomessy, and J. Neidecker

Five questions are most important when considering the selection of a prosthetic heart valve: hemodynamic performance, durability, thrombogenicity, prosthetic valve endocarditis and valve-induced intravascular hemolysis. Also taken into consideration are the type of substitute, the age and sex of the patient, and many other, particularly socio-economic implications.

With respect to the hemodynamic aspect of prosthetic heart valve replacement, we are faced with a large amount of published data on the different most widely implanted valves. Those are, in alphabetical order, the Björk-Shiley®, Lillehei-Kaster®, Starr-Edwards® and St. Jude Medical® valves for mechanical prostheses, and the Carpentier-Edwards, Hancock and Ionescu-Shiley bioprostheses. In an attempt to compare as comprehensively as possible the data gathered in the literature, we first have to consider the physical parameters of prosthetic valves, then in vitro hemodynamic studies of a particular valve and lastly comparative studies. The clinical data, harvested from early and late postoperative studies, will be subsequently analyzed according to the anatomic site of valvular implantation, mitral, tricuspid, and aortic. Our own data will be presented simultaneously.

Physical parameters of heart valve prostheses

Six main publications have been considered for the comparison of the valves being tested (1–6), as well as the data sheets provided by the manufacturers. The results computed in Table 1 show the actual dimensions of the prostheses collected in between orifice areas of the prostheses for a given tissue annulus diameter, so that the ratios between orifice area and tissue annulus area (O/A area) are found within rather wide limits. Considering the mechanical devices, the St. Jude Medical (SJM) valve shows the best ratios. Considering the bioprosthesis, the improved Carpentier-Edwards valve shows the best ratio in all sizes, in close relationship with the Ionescu-Shiley universal sewing ring prosthesis. This last model however shows a better ratio in the 19 mm size.

In vitro hemodynamic studies

Although far from reproducing the physiological strains which are applied on a prosthetic heart valve, the in vitro testing studies are a useful tool for assessing the characteristics of a prosthetic device and for comparing prostheses under the same conditions. Five main studies have been thoroughly reviewed to build a synthesis out of their conclusions (3, 5–8). The methodology followed by the various investigators is based on experiments conducted under both steady and pulsatile flow conditions within an artificial heart chamber. Steady flow testing is used to determine the transvalvular pressure gradient under static conditions,

Table 1. Physical parameters of various prosthetic heart valves. Abbreviations: B–S: Björk-Shiley, SJM: St. Jude Medical, L–K: Lillehei-Kaster, C–E: Carpentier-Edwards, HK: Hancock, ISU: Ionescu-Shiley univ. ring.

Valve	Tissue size	Annulus diam (mm)	Annulus area (cm²)	Orifice* diam (mm)	Orifice area (cm²)	O/A area
B–S	19	19	2.83	14	1.54	0.54
SJM	19	19	2.83	14.9	1.74	0.62
L–K	14A	19	2.84	14.2	1.54	0.54
C–E	19	19	2.83	18	1.84	0.65
HK	19		3.66	16	1.54	0.42
ISU	19	19	2.83	15.4	1.86	0.75
B–S	21	21	3.46	16	2.01	0.58
SJM	21	21	3.46	16.7	2.19	0.63
C–E	21	21	3.46	20	2.65	0.77
HK	21	21.6	4.37	18	2.01	0.46
ISU	21	21	3.46	17.4	2.38	0.69
B–S	23	23	4.15	18	2.54	0.61
SJM	23	23	4.15	18.67	2.74	0.66
C–E	23	23.2	4.22	22	3.50	0.83
HK	23	23.6	5.14	20	2.54	0.49
ISU	23	23	4.15	19.4	2.96	0.69
B–S	25	25	4.91	20	3.14	0.64
L–K	18M	25	4.91	18	3.1	0.63
SJM	25	25	4,91	20.5	3.30	0.67
SE 6120	1M	26	5.31	16.5	2.14	0.40
C–E	25	25.3	5.02	24	4.39	0.87
HK	25	25.6	6.02	21.8	3.80	0.63
ISU	25	25	4.91	21.4	3.60	0.73
B–S	27	27	5.72	22	3.8	0.66
SJM	27	27	5.72	22.6	4.01	0.70
C–E	27	27	5.72	25	4.68	0.82
HK	27	27.7	6.61	22	3.80	0.57
ISU	27	27	5.72	23.4	4.30	0.75
B–S	29	29	6.61	24	4.52	0.69
L–K	22M	29	6.61	22	3.80	0.57
SJM	29	29	6.61	24.3	4.64	0.70
SE 6120	3M	30	7.07	19.25	2.91	0.41
C–E	29	29.5	6.83	27	5.30	0.78
HK	29	29	8.29	24.3	4.90	0.59
ISU	29	29	6.60	25.4	5.07	0.77
B–S	31	31	7.54	24	4.52	0.60
SJM	31	31	7,54	26.2	5.39	0.71
C–E	31	31	7.54	28	6.16	0.81
ISU	31	31	7.54	27.4	5.90	0.78
B–S	33	33	8.55	24	4.52	0.53
SJM	33	33	8.55	26	5.31	0.62
C–E	33	33	8.55·	31.3	6.98	0.82
HK		32.5				
ISU	33	33	8.55	29.4	6.79	0.79

* calculated as area $= \pi r^2$

whereas testing with a pulse duplicator using controlled stroke volumes and pulse rates allows for the collection of the following data:
- Flow rate studies that can be applied on steady flows, root mean square flows, peak flows or mean flows (3);
- Effective orifice area (EOA), the computation of which uses the flow through the valve, the pressure gradient across it, and a discharge coefficient. This particular coefficient is mainly based on the planimetric orifice study of a given prosthesis;
- Performance index, representing the product of the discharge coefficient and the ratio of the actual valve orifice area to mounting area;
- Regurgitant flow through the prosthesis.

The four steady flow studies compare different devices of different sizes under different flow patterns and conditions, so that any type of synthesis between their conclusions may be invalid. The pulsatile flow studies on the other hand permit some stronger comparison. The pressure drop curves however cannot be compared from one author to the other since there may be some bias due to the different designs of the duplicators. Moreover, the type of flow utilized for establishing the curves is not always indicated (peak, steady, mean or root mean square flow), and the more extensive study (3) does not include the latest devices. The only valid comparisons were made between effective orifice areas (EOA) and performance

Table 2. Effective orifice area (EOA), performance index (PI), and discharge coefficient (DC) values based on the root mean square flow method.
Abbreviations: see Table 1.

Valve	EOA (cm^2)	PI	DC	Regurgitant vol. (ml/beat)
L–K 14A	1.13	0.40	0.73	–
ISU 19	1.26	0.44	0.67	–
B–S 21	1.30–1.54	0.37–0.45	0.64	5.5
SJM 21	2.08	0.60	0.60	7.6
C–E 21	1.05	0.30	–	–
ISU 21	1.49	0.43	–	–
HK 19	0.90	0.35	0.56	–
B–S 25	2.37	0.48	0.70	7.3
L–K 18M	1.55	0.32	0.61	–
SJM 25	3.23	0.66	0.66	9.7
S–E 1M	1.56	0.29	0.73	5.0
C–E 25	1.52	0.31	–	–
ISU 25	1.93	0.39	0.54	–
HK 23	1.64	0.32	0.54	–
B–S 27	2.59	0.45	–	8.5
SJM 27	4.05	0.71	–	10.6
S–E 2M	1.71	0.30	–	5.5
C–E 27	1.95	0.34	–	–
ISU 27	2.35	0.41	–	–
B–S 29	3.01	0.46	0.67	–
L–K 22M	2.67	0.40	0.70	–
S–E 3M	1.92	0.27	0.66	–
HK 27	1.98	0.30	0.52	–
IAU 29	2.96	0.45	0.58	–

Table 3. Average ventriculo-aortic peak systolic gradients, (mm Hg) in comparative postoperative hemodynamic studies after aortic valve replacement with various prostheses of different tissue annulus diameters.
Numbers in parentheses: gradient values with exercise.
NA = non–available data. * = early postoperative study.

Valve	Ref. no.	Tissue annulus diameter of aortic valve prosthesis									
		19		21		23		25		27	
B–S	(9)	–				18.9	(28.5)	15.6	(22.8)		
B–S	(10)	16	(NA)								
B–S	(14)*					12.3	(13.7)	13	(12.2)		
SJM	(9)					9.6	(15.7)	7.7	(11.7)		
SJM	(11)*	7.2	(15.1)	5.8	(14)	5.4	(12.4)	3.5	(8.7)		
SJM	(12)	16.7	(32)	0	(NA)						
SJM	(13)*			5.2	(3)	3.2	(3.6)	3.4	(3)		
SJM	(14)*			11	(13.5)						
SJM	(15)	6	(NA)	2	(NA)	2.4	(NA)	0.5	(NA)		
SJM	(16)	11	(NA)	9	(NA)	1.6	(NA)	2.07	(NA)	0	
L–K	(17)	45	(NA)	28	(NA)	22	(NA)	15	(NA)	5	(NA)
S–E	(17)	29	(NA)	18	(NA)	13	(NA)	21	(NA)	13	(NA)
C–E	(20)					7.6	(NA)	8.3	(NA)	6.6	(NA)
HK	(20)					10.8	(NA)	11.9	(NA)	11	(NA)
ISU	(21)	0	(4)			8.9	(11.7)	3.2	(10)		
ISU	(22)	12	(9)	6	(15)						

indices (PI). The results are collected in Table 2, along with values of the regurgitant flow expressed in ml/beat at a heart rate of 70/min (5). The data indicate that the St. Jude Medical valve in the size range of 21 to 27 on average has the best performance index, meaning that the resistance to flow through this prosthesis is even less than that through the tissue valves under study. It should be mentioned that the Carpentier-Edwards bioprosthesis is not the "improved" model. The data also indicate that the St. Jude Medical valve has a higher regurgitant flow than the corresponding mechanical valves. This has been partly explained by the asynchronous closure of the two leaflets (5, 9).

In vivo hemodynamic studies

There is an enormous amount of data regarding the hemodynamic evaluation of the prosthetic valves currently in use, but the reproducibility of the hemodynamic condition is rather poor from one study to the other, often precluding any valid conclusions to be drawn. The data computed in Tables 3 to 6 may seem incomplete but only truly comparable data have been kept for comparison. The aortic and mitral "situations" are separated for the analysis. Along with the "late" postoperative studies, some early studies are included, generally performed within 48 hours of surgery. Amongst them, our own study (14), still in process, is concerned with a comparison between Björk-Shiley and St. Jude Medical valves in the small aortic root using the sizes 19 and 21 mm at rest and with exercise simulated by atrial pacing and preloading. One of the conclusions to be drawn from Table 3 is that if the aortic annulus can accomodate a size 23 mm and above prosthesis, the peak systolic transvalvular gradient will never exceed 19 mm Hg at rest, and 28 mm Hg with exercise,

Table 4. Average mean diastolic gradient (mm Hg) accross prosthetic valves with different tissue annulus diameters after mitral valve replacement. Numbers in parentheses: transmitral gradients with exercise.

Valve	Ref. no.	Tissue annulus diameter of mitral valve prosthesis			
		25	27	29	31
B–S	(9)	–	–	4.5 (NA)	
B–S	(23)	–	6.2 (17.6)	6.2 (17.6)	
SJM	(9)	–	–	2.3 (NA)	
SJM	(13)*	1.4 (6.2)	1.9 (2.8)	1.8 (3.2)	1.6 (3.3)
SJM	(15)	–	2 (NA)	1 (NA)	0 (NA)
SJM	(16)	2.8 (NA)	1.8 (NA)	1.28 (NA)	2.2 (NA)
L–K	(17)	–	8 (NA)	8 (NA)	5 (NA)
S–E	(17)	10 (NA)	8 (NA)	10 (NA)	5 (NA)
C–E	(18)	–	7.1 (15)	7.1 (15)	5.1 (12)
C–E	(20)	–	2.8 (NA)	2.6 (NA)	2.1 (NA)
HK	(20)	–	3.7 (NA)	3.5 (NA)	3.2 (NA)

except for the Lillehei-Kaster valve. This is true for either mechanical or biological prostheses. The problems arise for the small aortic annulus, unable to accomodate prostheses larger than 19 or 21. In this regard, the 19 and 21 mm St. Jude Medical valves compare very favorably with the other devices due to a better effective orifice area at rest and with exercise (Table 5).

Table 5. Comparative calculated effective orifice areas (Gorlin) (cm^2) after aortic valve replacement.

Valve	Ref. no.	Tissue annulus diameter of aortic valve prosthesis				
		19	21	23	25	27
B–S	(9)	–	–	1.5 (1.9)	1.9 (2.1)	–
B–S	(10)	1.06 (NA)	–	–	–	–
B–S	(11)*	–	3.03 (NA)	2.07 (1,91)	3.51 (3.26)	3.57 (2.7)
SJM	(9)	–	–	2.2 (2.5)	2.6 (2.9)	–
SJM	(11)*	1.58 (1.44)	2.42 (1.98)	3.18 (2.4)	3.28 (4.43)	–
SJM	(12)	1.2 (1.1)	1.2 (1.1)	–	–	–
SJM	(13)*	–	2.7 (3.0)	3.6 (2.8)	3 (3.1)	–
SJM	(16)	1.38 (NA)	1.61 (NA)	2.32 (NA)	2.62 (NA)	3.67 (NA)
L–K	(17)	–	0.8 (NA)	1.1 (NA)	1.3 (NA)	1.9 (NA)
S–E	(17)	–	1.0 (NA)	1.1 (NA)	1.3 (NA)	1.8 (NA)
C–E	(18)	–	1.14 (1.28)	1.14 (1.28)	1.37 (1.57)	1.37 (1.57)
C–E	(20)	–	–	2.0 (NA)	2.3 (NA)	2.25 (NA)
HK	(19)*	–	1.59 (NA)	1.84 (NA)	1.95 (NA)	–
HK	(20)	–	–	1.8 (NA)	1.7 (NA)	2.2 (NA)
ISU	(21)	1.1 (1.4)	–	1.5 (2.1)	1.62 (2.03)	–
ISU	(22)	2.10 (1.5)	2.1 (1.5)	–	–	–

Table 6. Comparative calculated effective orifice areas (Gorlin) (cm^2) after mitral valve replacement.

Valve	Ref. no.	Tissue annulus diameter of mitral valve prosthesis			
		25	27	29	31
B–S	(9)	–	–	2.5 (2.8)	–
B–S	(23)	–	1.8 (2.2)	1.8 (2.2)	–
SJM	(9)	–	–	3.1 (3.4)	–
SJM	(13)*	2.1 (2.3)	2.1 (3.6)	2.8 (3.2)	3.1 (3.3)
SJM	(16)	3.0 (NA)	3.03 (NA)	3.36 (NA)	4.30 (NA)
L–K	(17)	1.1 (NA)	1.6 (NA)	1.7 (NA)	1.9 (NA)
S–E	(17)	1.4 (NA)	1.4 (NA)	1.4 (NA)	1.9 (NA)
C–E	(18)	–	2.33 (2.80)	2.33 (2.80)	2.68 (3.14)
C–E	(20)	–	–	3.0 (NA)	3.2 (NA)
HK	(20)	–	–	2.8 (NA)	3.0 (NA)

The results given in Table 4 show that the range of diastolic gradients accross a mitral prosthesis is obviously more narrow, even with exercise. In the most widely used sizes of 27 and 29 mm for the mitral valve replacement, the St. Jude Medical valve stays in the first position amongst the mechanical devices, again with a wider effective orifice area (Table 6).

Hemodynamics as a criterion for prosthetic valve selection

When it comes to the "weight" of hemodynamics for the selection of a prosthetic heart valve excluding all other criteria, it should be said first that both the hemodynamics of both the patient and the valve have to be taken into consideration.

The lack of genuine comparative studies between different prostheses has to be emphasized if one is concerned with hemodynamic performances. The post-operative evaluations should be reproducible and follow a rigid protocol, as recently advocated by Cohn (23). The latter however makes a complicated set-up mandatory and has to be carried out in the operation room shortly after the implantation of the prosthesis. The restrictions of this very peculiar hemodynamic situation are obvious.

In the aortic position, the main problem one has to deal with is the narrow aortic annulus. The two alternatives the surgeon is then faced with are either to proceed with a simple aortic valve replacement using a small size valve or to perform an aortic root enlargement procedure to gain one to three valve sizes. The corresponding risks are to leave a significant residual valvular gradient, or to increase the risks of the procedure which is often carried out, in our and others' experiences, in old women with heavily calcified aortic valves (10). In this situation, a 19 mm St. Jude Medical or Björk-Shiley valve may be the solution (10, 12). Care has to be taken of the body surface area of the patient (10): above 1.7 m^2, an aortic root enlargement of any type should be performed (10). Lastly, a patient's hemodynamic parameter can artificially lower a transvalvular gradient and should be considered at the time of implantation and at follow-up studies, namely, the left ventricular impairment.

In the mitral position, the patient's hemodynamics seems to be taking over the valve hemodynamics. Three conditions may drastically modify the outcome of the mitral valve replacement and hence determine the selection of a prosthesis: the presence of atrial fibrillation, a giant left atrium or a diminutive left ventricular cavity. Despite its somewhat higher regurgitant flow a prosthesis with a central flow and a favorable orifice to annulus ratio should be preferred (9).

In summary, the hemodynamic characteristics of a prosthetic heart valve are determinant and should be considered before any other criterion in two sets of circumstances:
- for an aortic valve replacement, in patients with a narrow aortic root, mainly if the body surface area is above 1.7 m^2;
- for a mitral valve replacement, in patients with either atrial fibrillation, giant left atrium, or small left ventricle.

References

1. Emery RW, Palmquist WE, Mettler E et al (1978) A new cardiac valve prosthesis: in vitro results. Trans Am Soc Artif Intern Organs 24:550
2. Brownlee RT, Walker DK, Scotten LN (1979) In vitro comparison of observed and calculated mitral valve area. Third International Symposium on artificial organs. Sao Paulo, Brazil
3. Gabbay S, McQeen DM, Yellin EL et al (1978) In vitro hydrodynamic comparison of mitral valve prostheses at high flow rates. J Thorac Cardiovasc Surg 76:771
4. Wright JT, Temple LJ (1971) An improved method for determining the flow characteristics of prosthetic mitral heart valves. Thorax 26:81
5. Yoganathan AP, Woo YR, Williams FP (1983) In vitro hydrodynamic characteristics of the St. Jude bileaflet aortic prosthesis. In: DeBakey ME (ed) Advances in Cardiac Valves. Yorke Medical Books, New York, p 229
6. Carpentier A, Dubost C, Lane E et al (1982) Continuing improvements in valvular bioprosthesis. J Thorac Cardiovasc Surg 83:27
7. Copeland JG, Larson DF, Lomen C et al (1982) Hemodynamics of the Ionescu-Shiley low profile aortic valve compared with other xenograft bioprostheses. Cardiac prosthesis symposium. Pebble Beach
8. Gabbay S, Yellin EL, Frishman WH et al (1980) In vitro hydrodynamic comparison of St. Jude, Björk-Shiley, and Hall-Kaster valves. Trans Am Soc Artif Intern Organs 26:231
9. Horstkotte D, Körfer R (1983) The influence of prosthetic valve replacement on the natural history of severe acquired heart valve lesions. In: DeBakey ME (ed) Advances in Cardiac Valves. Yorke Medical Books, New York, p 47
10. Schaff HV, Borkon AM, Hughes C et al (1981) Clinical and hemodynamic evaluation of the 19 mm Björk-Shiley aortic valve prosthesis. Ann Thorac Surg 32:50
11. Gray RJ (1983) Hemodynamic function of St. Jude aortic valves: comparison with a porcine and Björk-Shiley prostheses. In: De Bakey ME (ed) Advances in Cardiac Valves. Yorke Medical Books, New York, p 247
12. Wortham DC, Tri TB, Bown TE (1981) Hemodynamic evaluation of the St. Jude Medical valve prosthesis in the small aortic anulus. J Thorac Cardiovasc Surg 81:615
13. Chaux A, Gray RJ, Matloff JM et al (1981) An appreciation of the new St. Jude valvular prosthesis. J Thorac Cardiovasc Surg 81:202
14. Champsaur G, Gressier M. Ninet J et al (1984) Personal communication
15. Lillehei CW (1982) Worldwide experience with the St. Jude Medical valve prosthesis: clinical and hemodynamic results. Cardiovasc Med 1:309
16. Pyle RB, Mayer JE, Lindsay WG et al (1978) Hemodynamic evaluation of Lillehei-Kaster and Starr-Edwards prostheses. Ann Thorac Surg 26:336
17. Pelletier C, Chaitman BR, Baillot R et al (1982) Clinical and hemodynamic results with the Carpentier-Edwards porcine bioprosthesis. Ann Thorac Surg 34:612

18. Zusman DR, Levine FH, Carter JE et al (1981) Hemodynamic and clinical evaluation of the Hancock modified-orifice aortic bioprosthesis. Circulation 64 (Suppl II): 189
19. Levine FH, Carter JE, Buckley MJ et al (1981) Hemodynamic evaluation of Hancock and Carpentier-Edwards bioprostheses. Circulation 64 (Suppl II): 192
20. Tandon AP, Smith DR, Mary DA et al (1977) Sequential hemodynamic studies in patients having aortic valve replacement with the Ionescu-Shiley pericardial xenograft. Ann Thorac Surg 24:149
21. Bove EL, Helak JW, Potts JL et al (1982) Post-operative hemodynamic evaluation of the Ionescu-Shiley prosthesis in the small aortic root. Cardiac prosthesis symposium. Pebble Beach
22. Tandon AP, Sengupta SM, Lukacs L et al (1978) Long-term clinical and hemodynamic evaluation of the Ionescu-Shiley pericardial xenograft and the Braunwald-Cutter and Björk-Shiley prostheses in the mitral position. J Thorac Cardiovasc Surg 76:763
23. Cohn LH, Mudge GH, Gaspar J et al (1983) Hemodynamic evaluation of new cardiac valves. Ann Thorac Surg 35:359
24. Roberts WC, Bulkley BH, Morrow AG (1973) Pathologic anatomy of cardiac valve replacement: a study of 223 necropsy patients. Progr Cardiovasc Dis 15:539

Authors' address:
G. Champsaur, M. D.
Service de Chirurgie Cardiaque "C"
Hôpital Cardiologique Louis Pradel
59 Boulevard Pinai
69003 Lyon, France

Prosthetic Valve-related or Valve-induced Complications

D. Horstkotte and F. Loogen

All artificial heart valves are associated with a high rate of valve-related (mechanical dysfunction) or valve-induced complications (1,2). The *valve-related* complications can be direct consequences of hemodynamic disturbances persisting postoperatively (intravascular hemolysis), of the implanted artificial material (mechanical dysfunctions) or of both factors (prosthetic valve endocarditis, thrombosis of the prosthesis, thromboembolic events).

Those complications induced by the implantation of the prosthesis are mostly caused by the side effects of the necessary postoperative medical therapy, most frequently, bleeding related to anticoagulant therapy. Side effects of prophylaxis for valve-related endocarditis are very rare; but, because of high risk in all congenital and acquired heart valve failures, prophylaxis is almost always necessary even without valve replacement (3).

Although all these complications occur without mechanical malfunction of the prosthesis, their rate of occurrence is sometimes remarkably increased in cases of dysfunction of the prosthesis.

Chronic intravascular hemolysis (4) is today, with intact function of the prosthesis, of no clinical importance. However, hemolysis is still a very reliable parameter for measuring the extent of hemodynamic disturbance persisting postoperatively (5). The results published by Khayat in this volume also confirm the value of a graduation of hemolysis to detect prosthetic valve malfunctions and to show the relationship of prosthetic hemodynamics to the damage of corpuscular blood elements.

Recently, in the case of Ionescu-Shiley xenografts, toxic erythrocyte damage, mediated by the fixation medium glutaraldehyde, increased intravascular hemolysis (6).

In some cases, very high rates of hemolysis for mechanical prostheses, especially for the St. Jude Medical[R] prosthesis, have been reported without prosthetic malfunctions which could be hemodynamically evaluated. In one of our cases, a very small paravalvular leak of an aortic prosthesis, indicated both on angiography and auscultation, was verified intraoperatively. In this case, clinically untreatable hemolysis (LDH values of about 3,000 U/L) and chronically decreasing hemoglobin levels (to 8 g%) made reoperation necessary. In some cases with increased erythrocyte damage, minimal and hemodynamically irrelevant paravalvular leakages may therefore be responsible for high rates of hemolysis. Evidence that hemolysis is caused by changed flow characteristics, increased volume loss or an unusual adjustment of the prosthesis during implantation, can be verified by carefully restudying large patient groups without malfunction. In none of the prostheses did hemolysis exceed the statistical probability of the distribution (5).

The presumption that small paraprosthetic leakages produce more expressive erythrocyte damage than high regurgitation volumes, is consistent with current theories about hemodynamic causes of hemolysis: increased shearing forces in turbulent flow (7–9).

The fact that hemolysis is increased in patients with signs of heart failure and insufficiency murmurs does not necessarily contradict this presumption when the incidence of hemolysis is compared with those patients with murmurs only, as reported by Khayat. Furthermore, even invasive studies cannot prove whether an insufficiency murmur, which is angiographically correlated with a minimum of contrast medium regurgitation, is the result of an intraprosthetic regurgitation or a paraprosthetic leak with increased hemolysis.

Minimal regurgitation through a closed mechanical prosthesis (10) can be seen as, and is, a consequence of the construction principle sometimes (e.g. Smeloff-Cutter prostheses) distinctly expressed. This so-called "leakage flow" is meant to avoid platelet aggregation at places with low streaming velocities by a "washing effect". This is compatible with the intact function of the prosthesis. The total volume loss in relation to stroke volume, heart rate, prosthesis size and central pressure amounts to 2 to 12% of the forward volume (11, 12). Because of the 85° opening angle of the St. Jude Medical valve with leaflets standing parallel to the main stream direction (13), at very low cardiac output or during tachycardia this factor can lead to higher regurgitant fractions.

The quantification of hemolysis does not play a role in the indication for reoperation. Even with high hemolysis rates, persisting for years, consecutive pathological effects were not seen. The only criterion for reoperation, therefore, is a clinically noncompensated anemia.

In spite of considerable diagnostic progress and continuous efforts for an effective prophylaxis, prosthetic valve endocarditis is still a very severe complication after implantation of artificial heart valves. Although antimicrobial and operative therapies have been consequently improved, today we still have to expect a mortality of 30 to 70% in infections of prosthetic valves (14–16).

In general, early prosthetic valve endocarditis is a result of an infection acquired perioperatively and it is normally defined as occurring within 60 days postoperatively. However, there is no doubt that depending on the kind of germ, endocarditis occurring later can also be a consequence of a perioperative infection. In our patients, the frequency of early prosthetic valve endocarditis has decreased within the last few years, among other reasons, because of a prophylaxis with cefazoline. Between 1970 and 1974 the rate was a mean of 3% per year, and within the last few years it has decreased to less than 0.5%.

On the other hand, extensive statistical evaluation has so far shown no marked decreases in the frequency of late prosthetic valve endocarditis, which in our group was 0.6 events per 100 patient-years (17). With events occurring during the early postoperative period included, the cumulative rate of prosthetic valve endocarditis after 10 years amounts to 2.8% (17). The risk of endocarditis for mechanical valves is today estimated to be less than for biological valves (15, 18–21). The prognosis, however, is favorable for xenografts. If so-called early endocarditis is excluded, we found a cumulative prosthetic valve endocarditis rate of 2.5% over 15 years. This corresponds to a yearly incidence of about 0.17%, which is less than frequencies reported up to now (22,23).

The malfunctions caused by prosthetic valve endocarditis, including clinical and other findings, are summarized in this volume in the chapter "Incidence, Clinical Findings and Mangement of Prosthetic Valve Malfunction".

Prophylaxis is important to combat the high mortality (30% to 70%) of prosthetic valve endocarditis (24–26) because in patient groups with a particularly high risk for infection, the events causing the infection can be sufficiently defined and individual prophylaxes instituted (3).

After diagnostic or therapeutic interventions at the oropharynx or the respiration tract (27,28), bacteremia caused by streptococci is frequent. With the exception of flexible bronchoscopy without transbronchial biopsy, these manoeuvres, especially tooth extraction

Table 1. Bacteremia in diagnostic or therapeutic interventions

Oropharynx and dental/respiratory tract procedures

Tooth extraction	18–85%,	streptococci, hemophilus
Tonsillectomy	28–38%,	streptococci, hemophilus
Nasotracheal intubation	16%,	streptococci, staphylococci, gram-negative
Rigid bronchoscopy	15%,	bacilli
Flexible bronchoscopy	1%,	streptococci

Gastrointestinal and genito-urinary tract procedure

Genito-urinary surgery	7–82%,	gram. negative bacilli, enterococci
Cystoscopy	13–43%,	gram-negative bacilli
Gastro-duodenoscopy	4–13%,	staphylococci, diphtheroids
Contrast enema	12%,	gram-negative bacilli, enterococci
Coloscopy	6%,	coli, enterococci
Bladder catheterization	7%	
Normal delivery	0–5%,	streptococci and others

(According to Everett and Hirshman, 1977 (27) and Bisno, 1981 (28))

and other dental interventions leading to mucous membrane injuries require an endocarditis prophylaxis. For contrast enema, coloscopy and bladder catheterization, the documented frequency of bacteremia (mostly enterobacteria) occurs to such a degree that prophylaxis is also necessary. For uncomplicated deliveries, however, prophylaxis for endocarditis is regarded as not necessary (29) (Table 1).

Whether the recommended prohylaxis is actually used depends on the simplicity and practicability of its handling.

Recommendations of the American Heart Association (AHA) revised in 1984 (30), are based on the experimental studies of Durack (31) and advocate the use of bactericide-acting antibiotics. The original recommendations were used in recent years with various modifications.

A scheme for prophylaxis, based on the recommendations of the AHA, has been used at Düsseldorf (Tables 2 and 3); it has been proven effective in patients with prosthetic valve replacements, who are known as a high risk group for acquiring infective endocarditis.

Table 2. Prophylaxis for infective endocarditis in patients not allergic to penicillin

A. Bacteremia by "cocci" (dental procedures, diagnostic or therapeutic interventions at the oropharynx or the respiratory tract)
    60 minutes prior   2 ME penicillin G i.v.
                              + 1 g streptomycin i.m.*
    thereafter 24 h every 6 h (up to 48 h) 1 ME penicillin V orally

B. Bacteremia by "entero-bacteria" (abdominal surgery, gastrointestinal diagnostics, diagnostic and therapeutic procedures at the genito-urinary tract)
    60 minutes prior   1 g ampicillin i.v.
                              + 80 mg gentamicin i.v.
    after 8 h and 16 h repeated injections (up to 48 h)

*avoid i.m. injections in anticoagulated patients (e.g. use streptomycin-pantothenat)

Table 3. Prophylaxis for infective endocarditis in patients allergic to penicillin

A.	Bacteremia by "cocci" (dental procedures, diagnostic or therapeutic interventions at the oropharynx or the respiratory tract)

90 minutes prior   1.0 g erythromycin orally
thereafter 6 h every 6 h (up to 48 h)   0.5 g erythromycin orally

B.   Bacteremia by "entero-bacteria" (abdominal surgery, gastrointestinal diagnostics, diagnostic and therapeutic procedures at the genitourinary tract)

60 minutes prior   appr. 1.0 g cefolosporin i.m.*
                                              + 80 mg gentamicin i.v.

after 8 and 16 h repeated injections (up to 48 h)

* avoid i.m. injections in anticoagulated patients

Although it could not be documented that prophylaxis was consequently practised for all patients, 229 patients with 287 interventions and prophylaxis had no incidence of prosthetic valve endocarditis whereas 6 out of 304 patients without prophylaxis acquired prosthetic valve endocarditis. This corresponds to an incidence of 1.54 prosthetic valve infections per 100 interventions for patients without prophylaxis (3).

The practicability of this and other schemes for prophylaxis (32–34), has been criticized despite their obvious effectiveness, and the criticism is partially justified by the minimal use of these recommendations by physicians and patients.

Once it could be demonstrated that bactericidy is not an irreplaceable presupposition for an effective prophylaxis for endocarditis (36), simplified schemes for prophylaxis have recently been proposed (35).

Thromboembolic events and bleeding complications in patients needing anticoagulation represent the majority of complications after prosthetic heart valve replacement. The rate of thromboembolic events is still unsatisfactorily high, even after developing new prostheses with improved hemodynamics and new material which lessens thrombogenicity.

The thrombogenicity of mechanical heart valve prostheses, and to a lesser extent of biological heart valves, has most of all to be correlated with an activation of the thrombocytes (37), which is expressed in a reduced platelet survival time (38) and a release of thrombocyte specific enzymes such as β-thromboglobulin and platelet factor 4 which are able to initiate platelet aggregation. The platelet survival time is significantly lower after mitral, and especially after double valve replacement, than after aortic valve replacement. Corresponding to this, the risk of thromboembolism after double and mitral valve replacement is higher than after isolated aortic valve replacement.

Reduction of thrombocyte survival time and thrombus formation are supported by effects of turbulent flow on formed blood elements (37). These influences which consist of shearing forces and disintegration of blood elements are similar to those which, as a result of destruction of red blood elements, lead to hemolysis (37). Furthermore, the probability of thrombus formation at places of recirculation or blood stasis is increased. Because of the paraboloid flow profile, the velocity of the streaming through a heart valve is low and therefore the "washing effect" close to the valve ring is small. To prohibit platelet aggregation close to the valve ring, the majority of the prostheses used nowadays have a valve poppet which does not overlap the valve ring and therefore allows a mild regurgitation or "leakage flow" under closing conditions. Thus, because of the high streaming velocities, the adhesion of thrombus material will be prohibited. Whether this mechanism really antagonizes thrombus formation is questionable, because it could be demonstrated that high flows through small gaps can also support platelet aggregation (39). Additionally, leakage flow for some valve models means a considerable volume load on the ventricle.

The nearly central flow, almost complete absence of stasis downstream, and the use of highly polymerized pyrolytic carbon for the valve parts in the bloodstream, implicate the expectation of a low rate of thromboembolism for the St. Jude Medical valve (40, 41). Yet this prosthesis is not free from thromboembolic complications, and even thromboses of the valve have been reported (42).

Until endotheliazation is complete the sewing ring surface is also a source of thrombi. How thrombogenic valve housing and poppets made of metal or plastic material are is hard to quantify. Low rates of thromboembolism for valves with pyrolytic carbon (2, 41) seem to be possible because of the highly polished surface.

However, it is difficult to determine whether a thromboembolic event is related to the artificial valve or other factors, such as arrhythmia with atrial fibrillation, giant left atrium, etc.

The cumulative rate of thromboembolism 8 years after biological aortic valve replacement without anticoagulation is 1.8 to 4.3% (43). This corresponds to a frequency of 0.7 to 2.1 events per 100 patient-years. After mitral valve replacement, however, the incidence of thromboembolism (0.9 to 4.3 per 100 patient-years) (43) is nearly that of mechanical valves (0.7 to 1.9 events per 100 patient-years after aortic, and 0.9 to 4.6 events per 100 patient-years after mitral) (44, 45).

The manifestations of thromboembolic events are peripheral embolisms generated by the valve or thrombosis of the prosthesis. Thromboses of prosthetic heart valves are frequently above average in the tricuspid position, so that in many centers, xenografts are used for tricuspid valve replacement, if this is possible for hemodynamic reasons. Thromboses of the prostheses have been reported as sudden, often fatal events (46). However the majority of cases of valve thrombosis we have observed were progressing slowly. The loss of the opening or closing click of the prosthesis could be documented in all cases. The appearance of a new murmur and the loss of the valve opening or closing click, are important signs of a thrombosis, which in some cases occur before the patient becomes symptomatic.

Risk of thromboembolic events has to be compared with the risk of bleeding complications during lifelong anticoagulant treatment. Thromboembolic complications normally occur if the effect of the anticoagulation is not guaranteed (47). In 82% of our patients with thromboembolisms there was ineffective anticoagulation at the time of the event (Quick > 30%) (44). The majority of thromboembolic complications registered were associated with an interruption of anticoagulation because of minor interventions (e.g. tooth extraction).

Use of anticoagulants, however, puts a high responsibility on the physician and patient, not only because of thromboembolic risk with insufficient doses, but also because of severe, sometimes fatal, bleeding complications (48). More than one-third of all patients have a history of hemorrhagic complications within the first two postoperative years. Severe bleeding complications appear with a frequency of 1.8 to 4.4 per 100 patient-years (44).

The risk of thromboembolism can be reduced by combining anticoagulation and platelet aggregation inhibitors (49,50) but this combination risks a higher rate of severe bleeding complications (51). We cannot recommend such a combined therapy.

Mechanical dysfunctions of xenografts must be expected regularly after 8 to 15 years, in a frequency depending on the type of prosthesis and patients' individual parameters. Mechanical dysfunctions are rare in mechanical prostheses used today. Excluding a few series, the frequency is below 0.1%.

References

1. Silver MD (1979) Late complications of prosthetic heart valves: a pathologist's viewpoint. Am Heart J 88: 668.
2. Horstkotte D, Körfer R, Seipel L et al (1983) Late complications in patients with Björk-Shiley and St. Jude Medical heart valve replacement. Circulation 68 (Suppl II): 175
3. Horstkotte D, Rosin H (1984) Therapy and prophylaxis of infective endocarditis. Schw Med Wsch 144: 1575
4. Gehrmann, G, Bleifeld W, Loogen F (1966) Mechanische Hämolyse nach Implantation künstlicher Herzklappen. Z Kreislaufforschung 55: 25
5. Horstkotte D, Aul C, Seipel L et al (1983) Influence of valve type and valve function on chronic intravascular hemolysis following mitral and aortic valve replacement using alloprostheses. Z Kardiol 72: 119
6. Schistek R, Benzer A, Scharfetter H et al (1984) Toxic complication after implantation of aortic valves. Life Supp Syst, Proceeding XIth. Ann Meeting ESAO: 63
7. Crexells C, Aerichide N, Bonny Y et al (1972) Factors influencing hemolysis in valve prostheses. Am Heart J 84: 161
8. Sallam IA, Show A, Bain WH (1976) Experimental evaluation of mechanical hemolysis with Starr-Edwards, Kay-Shiley, and Björk-Shiley valves. Scand J Thorac Cardiovasc Surg 10: 117
9. Horstkotte D, Haerten K, Leuner Chr et al (1978) Chronic intravascular hemolysis following mitral valve replacement with Björk-Shiley, Lillehei-Kaster, and Starr-Edwards prostheses Z Kardiol 67: 629
10. Gentle CR (1982) Characterisation of leakage flow in cardiac valve prostheses. Life Supp Syst, Proceedings IXth, Ann Meeting ESAO: 102
11. Bellhouse BJ, Bellhouse FH (1976) Fluid mechanic performance of five prosthetic mitral valves. In: Kalmanson D (ed) The mitral valve: A pluridisciplinary approach. Arnold, London p 247
12. Levang OW, Levorstad K, Honglend T (1980) Aortic valve replacement. A nonrandomized study comparing the Björk-Shiley and Lillehei-Kaster disc valves. Scand J Thorac Cardiovasc Surg 14: 7
13. Dellsperger KC, Wieting DW, Baehr DA et al (1983) Regurgitation of prosthetic heart valves: Dependence on heart and cardiac output. Am J Cardiol 51: 321
14. Richardson JV, Karp RB, Kirklin JW et al (1978) Treatment of infective endocarditis: A 10-year comparative analysis. Circulation 58: 589
15. Watanakunakorn C (1979) Prosthetic valve endocarditis. Progr Cardiovasc Dis 22: 181
16. Dismukes WE (1981) Prosthetic valve endocarditis: Factors influencing outcome and recommendations for therapy. In: Bisno AL (ed) Treatment of infective endocarditis. Grune and Stratton, New York, London, Toronto, p 167
17. Horstkotte D, Körfer R, Loogen F et al (1984) Prosthetic valve endocarditis: Clinical findings and management. Eur Heart J 5 (Suppl C): 117
18. Johnson WD (1976) Prosthetic valve endocarditis In: Kaye D (ed) Infective Endocarditis. Univ Park Press, Baltimore, p 129
19. Arnett EN, Kastl DG, Garvin AJ et al (1977) A conversation on prosthetic valve endocarditis. Am Heart J 93: 510
20. Magilligan DJ, Quinn EL, Davila JC (1977) Bacteremia endocarditis and the Hancock valve. Ann Thor Surg 24: 508
21. Ferrans VJ, Boyce SW, Billingham ME et al (1979) Infection of glutaraldehyde-preserved porcine valve heterografts. Am J Cardiol 43: 1123
22. Madison J, Wang K, Gobel FL et al (1975) Prosthetic aortic valvular endocarditis. Circulation 51: 940

23. Masur H, Johnson WD (1980) Prosthetic valve endocarditis. J Thor Cardiovasc Surg 80: 31
24. Karchmer AW, Dismukes WE, Buckley MJ (1978) Late prosthetic valve endocarditis: Clinical features influencing therapy. Am J Med 64: 199
25. Richardson JV, Karp RB, Kirklin JW et al (1978) Treatment of infective endocarditis: A 10 year comparative analysis. Circulation 58: 589
26. McAnulty JH, Rahimtoola SH (1979) Surgery for infective endocarditis. JAMA 242: 77
27. Everett ED, Hirshman JV (1977) Transient bacteremia and endocarditis prophylaxis: A review. Medicine 56: 61
28. Bisno AL (1981) Antimicrobial prophylaxis of infective endocarditis. In: Bisno AL (ed) Treatment of infective endocarditis. Grune and Stratton, New York, p 281
29. Sugure D, Blake S, Tray P, MacDonald D (1980) Antibiotic prophylaxis against infective endocarditis after normal delivery – is it necessary? Br Heart J 44: 499
30. Shulman ST, Amren DP, Bisno AL et al (1984) Prevention of bacterial endocarditis. A statement for health professionals by the Committee on rheumatic fever and infective endocarditis of the Council on cardiovascular disease in the young. Circulation 70: 1123
31. Durack DT, Beeson PB, Petersdorf RG (1973) Experimental bacterial endocarditis III. Production and progression of the disease in rabbits. Br J Exp Pathol 54: 142
32. Brooks SL (1980) Survey of the compliance with the American Heart Association guidelines for the prevention of bacterial endocarditis. J Am Dent Assoc 101: 41
33. Hashway T, Stone LJ (1982) Antibiotic prophylaxis of subacute bacterial endocarditis for adult patients by dentists in Dade County, Florida. Circulation 66: 1110
34. Petersdorf RG (1978) Antimicrobial prophylaxis of bacterial endocarditis. Prudent caution or bacterial overkill? Am J Med 65: 220
35. Working Party of the British Society for Antimicrobial Chemotherapy (1982) The antibiotic prophylaxis of infective endocarditis. Lancet 1982/II: 1323
36. Glauser MP, Bernard JP, Moreillon P et al (1983) Successful single-dose amoxillin prophylaxis against experimental streptococcal endocarditis: Evidence for two mechanisms of protection. J Infect Dis 147: 568
37. Stein PD, Sabbah HN (1974) Measured turbulence and its effect on thrombus formation. Circulation Res 35: 608
38. Steele PP, Weily HS, Davies H et al (1975) Platelet survival time following aortic valve replacement. Circulation 551: 358
39. Rieger H (1976) Zur Physiologie und Pathophysiologie der Blutplättchen unter rheologischen Aspekten. Habil RWTH Aachen
40. Emery RW, Nicoloff DM (1979) St. Jude Medical cardiac valve prosthesis. In vitro studies. J Thor Cardiovasc Surg 78: 269
41. Horstkotte D, Haerten K, Herzer JA et al (1981) Preliminary results in mitral valve replacement with the St. Jude Medical prosthesis: Comparison with the Björk-Shiley valve. Circulation 64 (Suppl I): 203
42. Nunez L, Iglesias A, Stillo J (1980) Entrapment of leaflet of St. Jude Medical cardiac valve prosthesis by miniscule thrombus: Report of two cases. Ann Thorac Surg 29: 567
43. Cohn LH (1979) Bioprosthetic cardiac valves – anticoagulation or not? In: Sebening F et al (eds) Bioprosthetic cardiac valves. Deutsches Herzzentrum, Munich, p 107
44. Horstkotte D, Körfer R, Budde Th et al (1983) Late complications following Björk-Shiley and St. Jude Medical heart valve replacement. Z Kardiol 72: 251
45. Horstkotte D, Haerten K, Herzer JA et al (1983) Five-year results after randomized mitral valve replacement with Björk-Shiley, Lillehei-Kaster and Starr-Edwards prostheses. Thor Cardiovasc Surg 31: 206
46. Krausz Y, Appelbaum A, Halon DA et al (1977) Thrombosis on Björk-Shiley aortic valve prostheses. Case report and review of literature. Isr J Med Sci 13: 410
47. Fuster V, Pumphrey CW, McGoon MD et al (1982) Systemic thromboembolisms in mitral and aortic Starr-Edwards prostheses: A 10–19 year follow-up. Circulation 66 (Suppl I): 157
48. Loogen F, Horstkotte D (1982) Therapy of cardiovascular disease – valvular heart disease. In: Bleifeld W, Mathey D (eds) Therapy of Cardiovascular Disease. Thieme, p 21
49. Taguchi K, Matsumura H, Washizu T et al (1975) Effect of athrombogenic therapy, especially high dose therapy of dipyridamole, after prosthetic valve replacement. J Cardiovasc Surg 16: 8

50. Sullivan MJ, Harken DE, Gorlin R (1971) Pharmacologic control of thromboembolic complications of cardiac valve replacement. New Engl J Med 284: 1391
51. Dale J (1977) Prevention of arterial thrombosis with acetylsalicylic acid in patients with prosthetic heart valves. Thromb Haemostas 38: 66

Authors' address:
Dr. Dieter Horstkotte
Medizinische Klinik der
Universität Düsseldorf
Moorenstraße 5
4000 Düsseldorf
F.R.G.

Non-invasive Follow-up of Prosthetic Heart Valves

U. Sigwart and L. Finci

The ideal prosthetic heart valve should be non-obstructive, non-thrombogenic, durable and silent.

Unfortunately, these features have not been achieved to date despite considerable progress in design and construction of prosthetic heart valves. Durability is still the main problem in tissue valves and thromboembolism is the predominant concern after implantation of mechanical valves. Therefore, routine functional control of the status of an artificial valve should be performed in every patient, even in the absence of particular problems.

Before suspecting malfunction, it is important that the physician be aware of the different categories of valve models and their normal findings with regard to their particular design. At the present time, there are five design categories of prosthetic heart valves; central ball occluder valves, central disc occluder low profile valves, excentric monocuspid tilting disc valves, bileaflet prostheses, and xenografts.

Ball valves

For historic reasons, ball valves have the longest proven durability; they also remain the standard for comparison. Typical examples are the Starr-Edwards® and the Smeloff-Cutter valve. They tend to have relatively high transvalvular gradients (1). The thromboembolic risk is estimated to be 2.9 to 6.4% per patient year (2).

Low profile disc valves

The advantages of low profile disc valves are certainly overestimated. The low profile was felt to be desirable in both the mitral and the aortic positions. However, large gradients across the centrally located disc occluder hindered the widespread use of this type of valve (3). A well known representative of this design is the Beall® prosthesis, the failure rate of which is significant due to disc wear (4). The incidence of thromboembolisms and hemolysis is comparable with ball valves.

Tilting disc valves

A widely used tilting disc valve is the Björk-Shiley® valve followed by the Lillehei-Kaster® and the Hall-Medtronic® valve. All tilting disc valves allow the disc occluder to pivot between 60 and 80° from the closed position just providing a near central flow. The obstruction to forward blood flow in tilting disc valves is somewhat lower than in ball valves (5), but thromboembolism continues to be a problem. Thrombosis of the valve can occur rapidly and may represent a real emergency situation (6).

Bileaflet disc valve

Bileaflet heart valves, the prototype of which is the St. Jude Medical® valve, are now copied by other manufacturers. In the open position, the leaflets are about parallel to the direction of the blood stream. Together with the favourable orifice to tissue annulus ratio the transprosthetic gradients appear to be lower than in any other comparable prosthetic heart valve (1,7,8). So far the St. Jude Medical valve appears to be durable and the incidence of thromboembolic events compares favourably with valves of other designs (9). Its major potential disadvantage is the delicate suspension of the parallel pivots which allow the leaflets to open up to 85° from the closed position and to fall entirely within the orifice ring at 30 to 35°. Theoretically, the hinge mechanism can interfere more easily with mechanical damage or thrombus formation in it. With a low rate of mechanical dysfunctions and prosthetic thromboses in the mitral and aortic positions, even after implantation of numerous prostheses, the hinge of the St. Jude Medical valve has so far not proven to be an important cause of malfunctions within the implantation period followed up.

The copied bileaflet prostheses which have been implanted in only small patient groups must prove this, particularly since in these the hinge joint mechanism has been altered.

Xenografts

The main advantage of xenografts (porcine or pericardial bioprostheses) is the relatively low incidence of thromboembolic disorders (10) which make them the model of choice in patients with high risk of bleeding complications under anticoagulant therapy and especially in women who would like to have children. Their durability, however, is limited so that after about 8 years, sometimes even earlier, reoperation must be considered.

Routine examination of patients with prosthetic heart valves

The following should be checked each time a patient with an artificial heart valve is examined:
- function of mobile parts
- variance of mobile parts
- thrombus formation
- valvular dehiscence

The available tests for the clinical follow-up of artificial heart valves are (10):
- history and physical examination
- phono- and mechanocardiogram
- parameters indicating hemolysis
- echocardiogram
- Doppler ultrasound studies
- invasive studies including cardiac catheterization
- angiography

The function of mobile parts

A manifestation of malfunction of mobile parts should be suspected in reference to the implanted model. In ball valves, the central ball occluder moves rapidly between the open and closed positions producing a characteristic opening and closing sound.

In the aortic position, the opening click is normally loud and occurs 0.07 to 0.09 s after the first component of the first heart sound. In the mitral position, a prominent opening click is normally recorded 0.06 to 0.12 s following the aortic component of the second heart sound. Each variation of these limits leads to a suspicion of malfunction (12,13). In the aortic position, the poppet may produce multiple systolic clicks which are due to turbulent flow and the repetitive touching of the cage-struts by the poppet. These phenomena can be observed during fluoroscopy and are entirely normal.

With the exception of Smeloff-Cutter prostheses a regurgitant flow of ball valves is unusual and normally indicates malfunction of the moving part or valvular dehiscence. Normal valve function can be observed with fluoroscopy. Beside mobility and structural integrity, the motion characteristics of the occluder can be evaluated (14). Abnormal tilting movement of the base ring indicates valvular dehiscence.

High precision functional studies of the ball excursions can be obtained through high speed radiocinematography; it is possible to determine the exact center of the ball and to measure the displacement. The excursions should be in accordance with the specifications of the manufacturer. Unfortunately, the occluder in early ball valves was not coated with radiopaque material. Therefore, exact observation of the ball excursions is poor and requires special photographic techniques. Ball variance is no longer an essential problem (16) but thrombotic material will clearly limit the ball excursions (15).

The anterior and posterior surface of the ball can readily be recorded by echocardiography in both the aortic and mitral positions (13). The only problem is the determination of the access of the echo beam with respect to the ball.

Eccentric occluder valves show similar auscultatory findings to ball valves. In the mitral position, they produce a loud opening sound with an A2-mitral opening interval from 0.07 to 0.12 s (13,17). There are no systolic murmurs caused by this type when implanted in the mitral position, but a diastolic murmur produced by turbulent flow and obstruction to forward blood flow can frequently be heard. Any change of the intensity of the diastolic

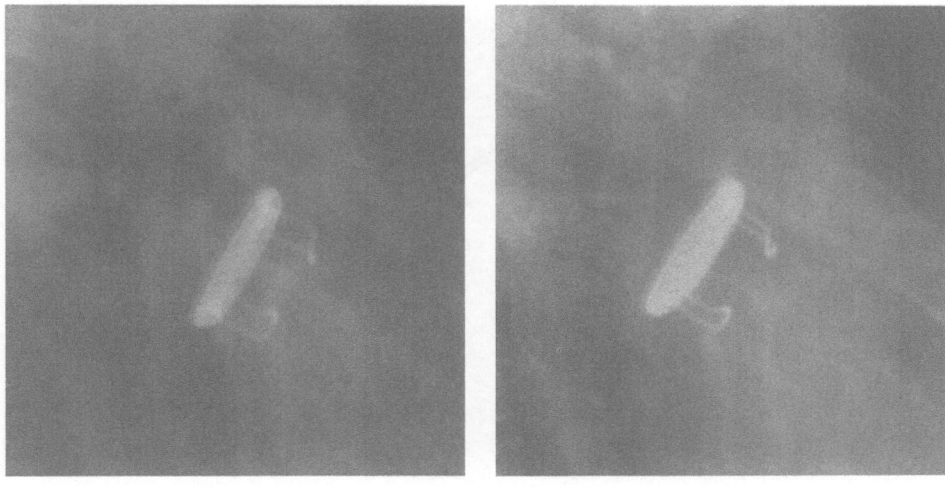

1a   1b

Fig. 1a and b. Central occluder disc valve showing intermittent dysfunction with incomplete closure (b).

murmur should alert the physician to suspect disc variance or malfunction. The best way to examine the correct performance of the central disc occluder is fluoroscopy and radiocinematography. Fig. 1 a and b gives an example of a low profile disc valve which opens correctly, but from time to time remains in systole at the lower edge of the disc, producing an incomplete closure. The reason for this is a thrombus formation, which can also be identified by abnormal movements of the occluder that can be seen with echocardiography (18, 19).

The variance of the mobile part

The first manifestation of ball variance may be a thromboembolic event. Therefore it is important to obtain the very specific patient history directed to possible thromboembolic problems. Auscultation of the heart helps in some instances but it is more important to perform a direct evaluation of the motion of the mobile parts by echocardiography.
Two-dimensional echocardiography (Fig. 2) allows us to follow the excursions of the mobile parts for a relatively long period of time. Due to its unlimited observation period, echocardiography seems to be more appropriate than fluoroscopy examinations for the detection of indefinite changes in normal poppet movement, especially if valve malfunction occurs only occasionally.
Ball or disc excursions are recorded by M-mode echocardiography, preferably under two-dimensional guidance. In the mitral position the eccentric monocuspid Björk-Shiley disc produces a brisk opening motion, a sharp E point and a prolonged EF slope. With the onset of ventricular systole the valve closes abruptly. In the aortic position, multiple echos can be recorded behind the left atrium. Two-dimensional echo is of minor value because of multiple reverberating echos arising from the suture ring and the disc. Cinefluoroscopy provides an excellent method for studying tilting disc valve motion (20). Figure 3 gives an example of the

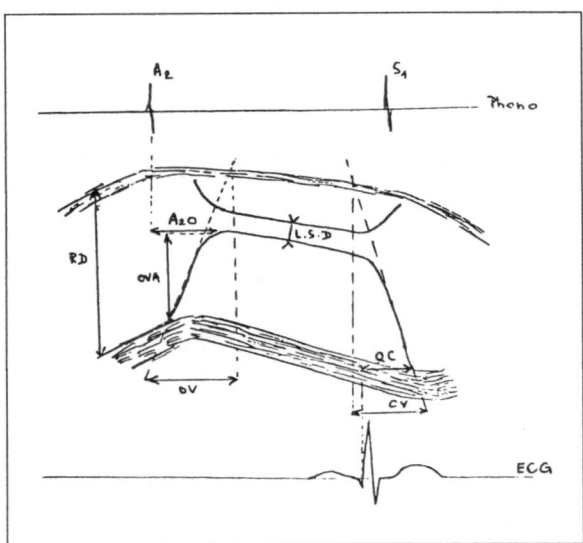

Fig. 2. Two dimensional echocardiography of a St. Jude Medical valve permitting timing of events and measurement of opening and closing characteristics (schematic).

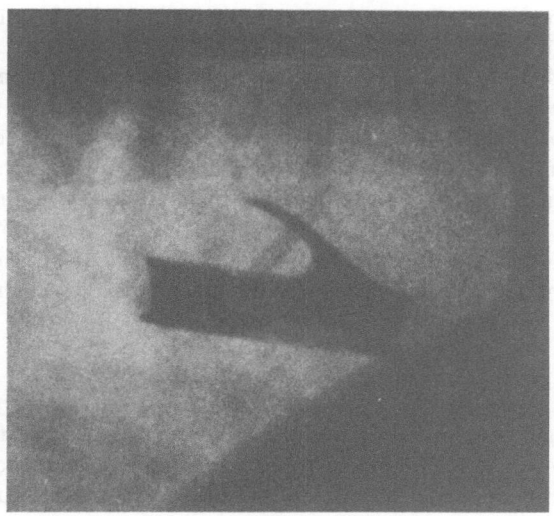

Fig. 3. A Lillehei-Kaster valve in the aortic position.

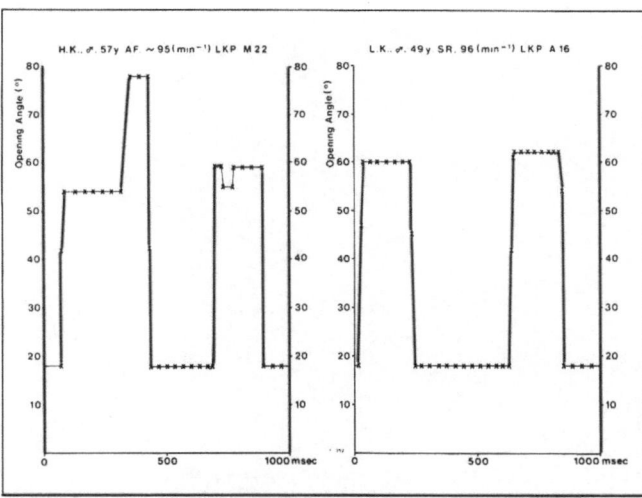

Fig. 4. Changes in the opening angle of Lillehei-Kaster valves due to turbulences. Reprinted from Sigwart et al. (20) with permission.

Lillehei-Kaster valve in the aortic position. During systole the disc is in an 80° position. For hemodynamic reasons this is not always the case. Turbulences may prevent the disc from opening fully to the design specification, as is demonstrated in Fig. 4. Patients with alterations of the hemodynamics, for instance in atrial fibrillation, may thus change their maximum opening angle from beat to beat (Fig. 4), which is not a sign of prosthetic valve malfunction, but of the hydrodynamic instability of the valve (20). The same is valid for the Björk-Shiley valve with the concave-convex designed disc, in which the effective opening angle in vivo is smaller than the technical opening angle (8). No hemodynamic advantage

91

was found in comparison to the Björk-Shiley Standard valve. Moreover, the increase in mechanical failures meant a definite step backwards.

The leaflet motions of the St. Jude Medical valve can be monitored with echocardiography in many instances (22,23). It must be assured, however, that the orientation of the valve is adequate for non-invasive follow-up. Cineradiography may also detect abnormal leaflet motion in cases where the X-ray beam can be directed parallel to the pivoting access of the disc occluders. Figure 5 shows an example of a St. Jude Medical valve in the mitral position. In Fig. 5a the valve is shown with an opening angle of 85° and in Fig. 5b it is closed at 35°. Figure 5c shows one leaflet in a half-open position, whereas the other is fully closed. The reason for this malfunction was thrombotic material which intermittently interfered with the normal closing mechanism.

Dehiscence and valvular regurgitation

In patients with paravalvular regurgitation, mitral or aortic regurgitation murmurs are usually heard. In some instances, however, despite the occurrence of significant paravalvular leaks, no murmur is audible. Clinical findings in advanced cases include severe anaemia due to increasing intravascular hemolysis (24) and heart failure. The echocardiographic signs include shortening of the interval between the second heart sound and the complete opening of the ball or disc, abnormal anterior motion of the disc just after full opening, abnormal left

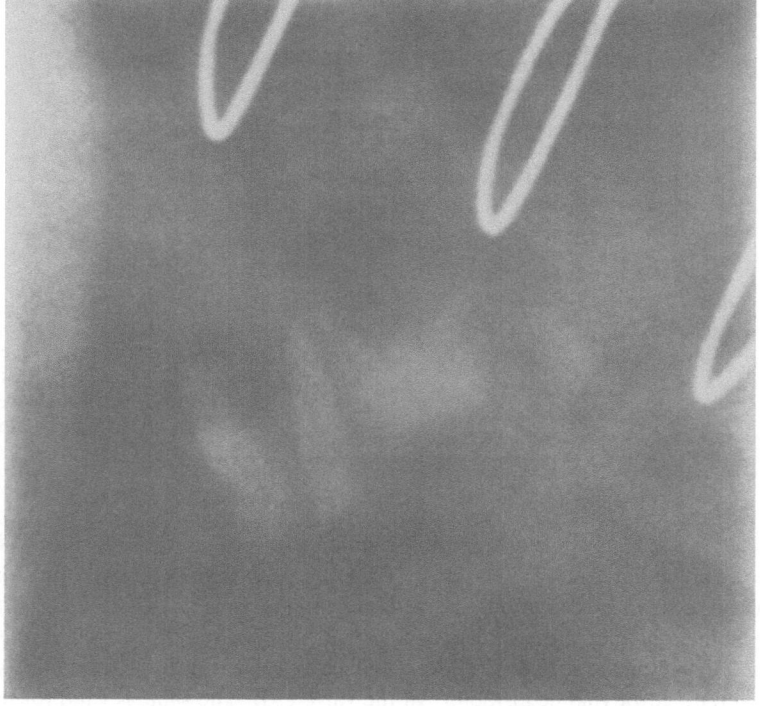

5a

Fig. 5a, b and c. St. Jude Medical valve in nitral position: a=open, b=closed. Occasionally (c) closure is incomplete due to thrombotic material.

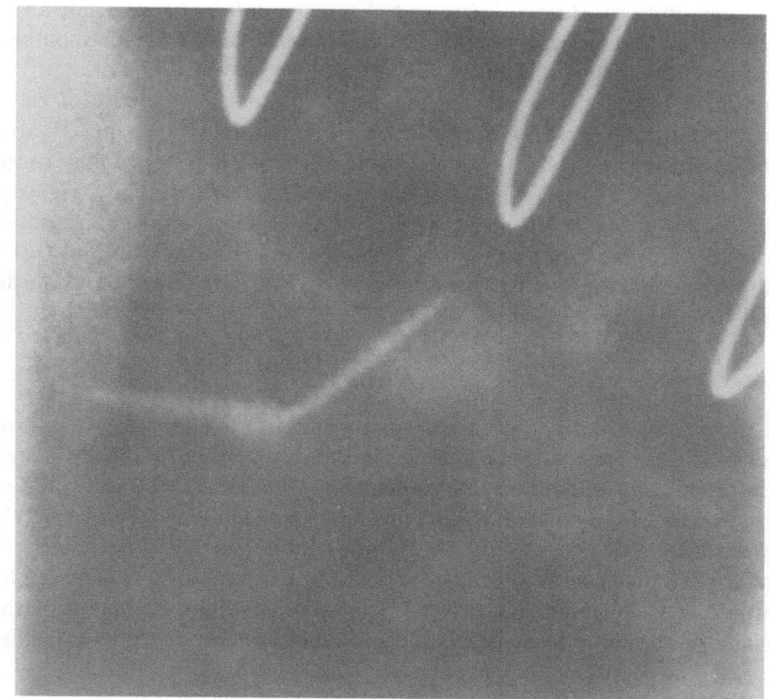

5b

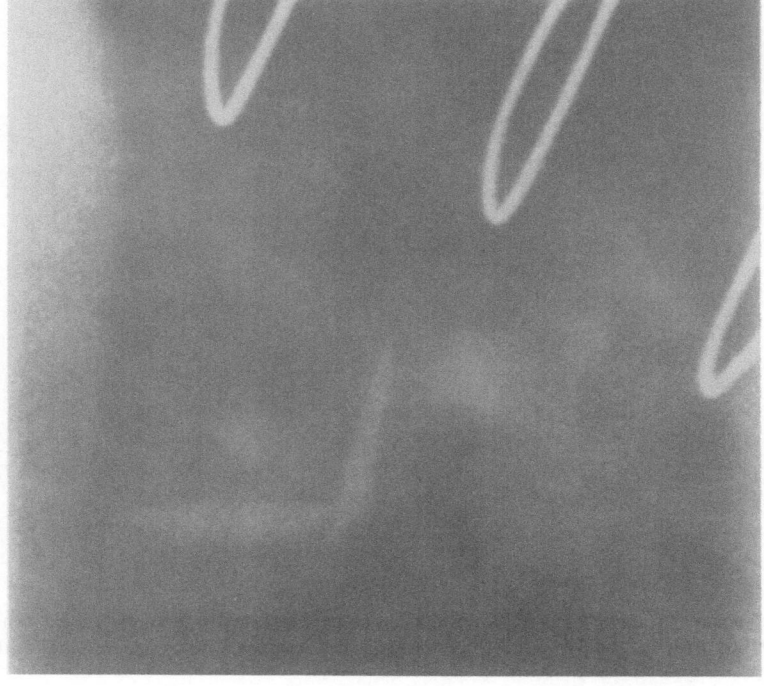

5c

ventricular wall motion, changes of peak rates, and changes in left ventricular left atrial diameters (12,19,25). These findings correlate well with periprosthetic regurgitation, but the specificity and sensitivity are unknown, and may persist after successful surgery.

Doppler ultrasound techniques can give information on the presence or absence of valve regurgitation. Quantifying the degree of regurgitation in the presence of a heart valve prosthesis however is difficult and sometimes impossible. A major dehiscence may cause striking abnormal motions of the prosthesis that can be recognized by fluoroscopy. Figure 6 shows a Lillehei-Kaster valve removed from a patient with subacute bacterial endocarditis. At the time of surgery, the valve could be removed without cutting a single suture. If the rocking movement of the valve ring is greater than 9 to 12° in mitral and 6 to 10° for aortic prostheses, paravalvular leaks must be suspected (26,27).

Prosthetic valve thrombosis

Auscultatory findings including the appearance or disappearance of opening and closure clicks and the change of the intensity of the murmurs can lead directly to the diagnosis of prosthetic valve thrombosis. In bioprostheses, the auscultatory findings may be non-specific. With echocardiography, clot formation or vegetations may be visualized directly (28,29). Alteration of the excursions of the moving parts, intermittent, incomplete or delayed opening with short intervals between the second heart sound and mitral valve opening due to flow obstruction are the most common features (13). The rounding of the E-point of mitral valve motion may indicate thrombus formation of the Björk-Shiley valve. In thrombosed St.

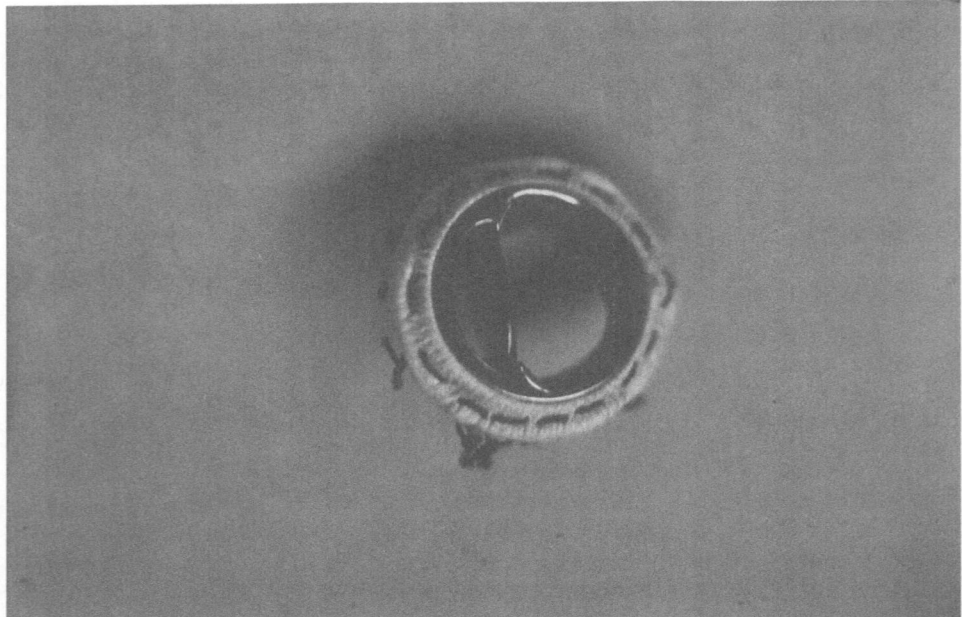

Fig. 6. Lillehei-Kaster valve, removed from the aorta without having to cut one single suture. The sewing ring was about to be dislodged due to subacute bacterial endocarditis. Diagnosis was made with fluoroscopy.

Jude Medical mitral leaflets the closing sound is diminished and the interval between second heart sound and mitral valve opening click is shortened. The best ways to control the integrity of poppet movement are fluoroscopy and cineradiography.

Adequate orientation of the prosthetic heart valve may be crucial for adequate non-invasive follow-up examinations. Therefore, cardiac surgeons should be aware of the difficulties in obtaining good echocardiographic and fluoroscopic visualization of the moving parts of artificial heart valves.

References

1. Horstkotte D, Haerten, K, Seipel L et al (1983) Central hemodynamics at rest and during exercise after mitral valve replacement with different prostheses. Circulation 68 (Suppl II): 161
2. McGoon D, Huster V, Punphrey C et al (1983) Aortic and mitral valve incompetence: Long-term follow-up (10 to 19 years) of patients treated with the Starr-Edwards prosthesis. JACC 3: 930
3. Reid JA, Stevens TW, Sigwart U et al (1972) Hemodynamics evaluation of the Beall mitral valve prosthesis. Circulation 45 (Suppl I): 1
4. Jost RG, McKnight RC, Roper CL (1975) Failure of Beall mitral valve prosthesis. J Thorac Cardiovasc Surg 70: 163
5. Horstkotte D, Haerten K, Körfer R et al (1983) Hemodynamic findings at rest and during exercise after implantation of different aortic valve prostheses. Z Kardiol 72: 429
6. Krausz Y, Appelbaum A, Halon DA et al (1977) Thrombosis on Björk-Shiley aortic valve prostheses. Case report and review of literature. Isr Med Sci 13: 410
7. Horstkotte D, Haerten, K, Herzer JA et al (1981) Preliminary results in mitral valve replacement with the St. Jude Medical prosthesis: Comparison with the Björk-Shiley valve. Circulation 64 (Suppl II): 203
8. Bruss KH, Reul H, van Gilse J et al (1983) Pressure drop and velocity fields at four mechanical heart valve prostheses: Björk-Shiley Standard, Björk-Shiley convex-concave, Hall-Kaster and St. Jude Medical. Life Supp Syst 1: 3
9. Horstkotte D, Körfer R, Budde Th et al (1983) Late complications following Björk-Shiley and St. Jude Medical heart valve replacement. Z Kardiol 72: 251
10. Minale C, Bardos P, Bourg NP et al (1982) Early and late results of porcine bioprostheses versus mechanical prostheses in aortic and mitral position. In: Cohn LH, Gallucci V, Cardiac bioprostheses (eds) Yorke Medical Books, New York, 1954
11. Horstkotte D, Loogen F (1983) Erfolgsbeurteilung mit invasiven und nichtinvasiven Methoden nach Herzklappenoperationen. Z Kardiol 72 (Suppl II): 16
12. Brodie BR, Grossman W, McLaurin L et al (1976) Diagnosis of prosthetic mitral valve malfunction with combined echo-phonocardiography. Circulation 53: 93
13. Katler MN, Mintz GS, Panidis I et al (1983) Noninvasive evaluation of normal and abnormal prosthetic valve function. JACC 2: 151
14. Sands MJ, Lachman AS, O'Reilly DJ et al (1982) Diagnostic value of cinefluoroscopy in the evaluation of prosthetic heart valve dysfunction. Am Heart J 104: 622
15. Hylen JC (1972) Mechanical malfunction and thrombosis of prosthetic heart valves. Am J Cardiol 30: 396
16. Hylen JC, Kloster FE, Starr A et al (1970) Aortic ball variance: Diagnosis and treatment. Ann Intern Med 72: 1
17. Bendt TB, Goodman DJ, Popp RL (1976) Echocardiographic and phonocardiographic confirmation of suspected mitral valve malfunction. Chest 70: 221
18. Copass H, Lakier JB, Kinsley RH et al (1980) Thrombosed Björk-Shiley mitral prosthesis. Circulation 61: 169
19. Bernal-Ramirez JA, Philipps JH (1977) Echocardiographic study of malfunction of Björk-Shiley prosthetic heart valve in the mitral position. Am J Cardiol 40: 449
20. Sigwart U, Schmidt H, Gleichmann U et al (1976) In-vivo evaluation of the Lillehei-Kaster heart valve prostheses. Ann Thorac Surg 22: 213

21. Horstkotte D, Haerten K, Schulte HD et al (1983) Hemodynamic findings at rest and during exercise after implantation of different mitral valve prostheses with equal tissue annulus diameter. Z Kardiol 72: 385
22. Amann FW, Burckhardt D, Hasse J et al (1981) Echocardiographic features of the correctly functioning St. Jude Medical valve prosthesis. Am Heart J 101: 45
23. Feldman HJ, Gary RJ, Chaux A et al (1982) Non-invasive in vivo and in vitro study of the St. Jude mitral valve prosthesis. Evaluation using two-dimensional M-mode echocardiography, phonocardiography and cinefluoroscopy. Am J Cardiol 49: 1101
24. Horstkotte D, Aul C, Seipel L et al (1983) Influence of valve type and valve function on chronic intravascular hemolysis following mitral and aortic valve replacement using alloprostheses. Z Kardiol 72: 119
25. Agnew TM, Carliste R (1970) Premature valve closure in patients with a mitral Starr-Edwards prosthesis and aortic incompetence. Br Heart J 32: 436
26. White AF, Dinsmore E, Buckley MJ (1973) Cineradiographic evaluation of prosthetic cardiac valves. Circulation 48: 882
27. Gahl K, Lücke R, Trost A et al (1979) Bewegungsspiel und Hämolysegrad von Herzklappenprothesen. Med Klinik 74: 909
28. Dillon JC, Feigenbaum H, Konecke L et al (1973) Echocardiographic manifestation of valvular vegetations. Am Heart J 86: 698
29. Ben-Zwi J, Hildner FJ, Chandraratna et al (1974) Thrombosis on Björk-Shiley aortic valve, prosthesis: clinical, arteriographic, echocardiographic and therapeutic observation in seam cases. Am J Cardiol 34: 538

Authors' address:
U. Sigwart, M.D.
Division of Cardiology
Department of Medicine
Centre Hospitalier Universitaire Vaudois
CH-1011 Lausanne
Switzerland

Hemolysis Following Cardiac Valve Replacement

M. C. Khayat, J. Piard, C. Zerr and A. Khayat

Destruction of red blood cells is a well-known phenomenon after heart valve replacement. Since the first description, clinically significant hemolysis has continuously decreased as a result of the progress in materials and the improved hemodynamic design of prostheses.

Chronic intravascular hemolysis after heart valve replacement

Over a 4-year period (1980–1983), hemolysis data were determined for this study in 591 patients. Parameters were determined postoperatively at the third month, the first year and the second year. The presented results are from the evaluation at the third month postoperative. Types and positions of valve prosthesis are shown in Table 1. Patients were separated into 3 groups. The first group includes 517 patients with single or double valve replacement without paravalvular leaks. The second group includes 46 patients with periprosthetic leaks separated into patients with only a valvular murmur (n=22) and patients with a murmur and associated cardiac failure (n=24). To assess the validity of laboratory tests taken after cardiac surgery, 28 patients undergoing coronary surgery were evaluated as a control group.

Laboratory tests for evidence of hemolysis were performed in all patients. The usual tests were: red cell count (erythrocytes), reticulocytes and shistocytes; hemoglobin concentration, free plasma hemoglobin; platelet count; serum lactic dehydrogenase activity (LDH); haptoglobin; hemopexin; serum iron and total iron binding capacity; and serum bilirubin. Urinary tests were done for hemoglobin and hemosiderin. The normal ranges (mean $\pm$ 2 standard deviations) for our laboratory unit are shown in Table 2. Statistical analysis was carried out by the chi-square method to compare capital frequencies, and by Student's test for mean values. Relationships between different tests were evaluated by correlation curves on 6 standard biological equations ($y=ax+b$; $y=1(a/x+b)$; $y=a\sqrt{x}+b$; $y=x^a+b$; $y=a$ log $x+b$). For statistical significance, the p value was estimated from the non-significant level (NS : $p \geq 0.05$) up to 10^{-12}. According to hemolysis data, the best correlation curves were selected at the lowest p values.

Table 1. Types and position of valvular implants

- Starr-Edwards (1260–6120)
- Björk-Shiley (aortic)
- Lillehei-Kaster (aortic)
- Omniscience (aortic)
- St. Jude Medical (aortic and mitral)
- Hall-Kaster (aortic)
- Carpentier-Edwards (aortic and mitral)
- Miscellaneous

Table 2. Normal range of laboratory test (mean ± standard deviation)

Erythrocytes	.4.6 ± 0.8 M/ml
Reticulocytes	38000 ± 32000/ml
Shistocytes	(class determination)
LDH	180 ± 60 U/l
Haptoglobin	1.1 ± 0.5 g/l
Hemopexin	0.8 ± 0.3 g/l
Bilirubin	9.5 ± 7.5 umol/l

Quantification of chronic intravascular hemolysis

According to the mechanism of intravascular hemolysis, the LDH level is directly correlated to the destruction of erythrocytes and LDH seems to be the prototypic parameter indicating red cell damage. Nevertheless, its sensitivity is not so sharp and, in the usual biological range of hemolysis, it is difficult to separate the characteristics of the different valvular implants. All other tests are multicorrelated with hemolysis and the sensitivity of the test varies with the level of red cell damage in a non-linear correlation curve.

The correlation between haptoglobin and LDH is the most characteristic example for this non-linear relationship of different levels of sensitivity (Fig. 1). The curve shows an excellent sensitivity of the haptoglobin test even in subclinical hemolysis rates and allows separation of the degrees of hemolysis after implantation of different types of prosthesis. However, haptoglobin levels are influenced by the inflammation which is usually present in the first weeks after surgery. The correlation between haptogobin values and inflammation (orosomucoid protein) is shown in Fig. 2 for Carpentier-Edwards xenografts and the control group. The correlation curve between hemopexin and LDH (Fig. 3) indicates a higher level

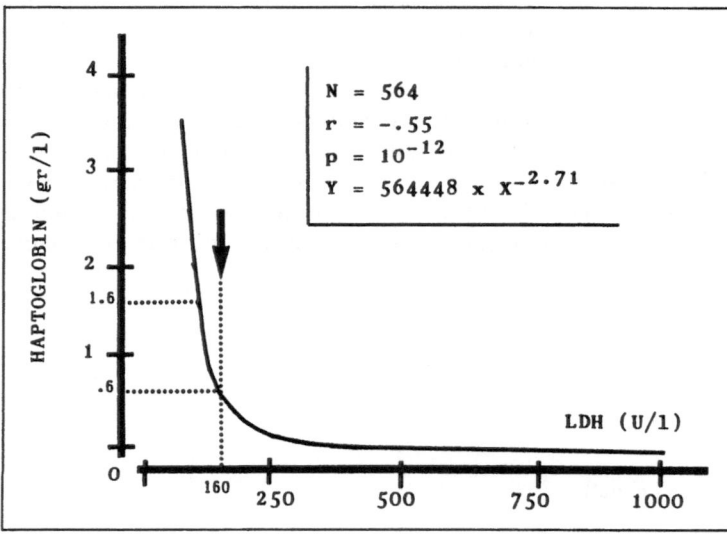

Fig. 1. Correlation curve between haptoglobin and LDH. Dotted lines and arrow indicate the normal range and limits of the tests. Sensitivity of the haptoglobin test is highest under 250 u/l of LDH.

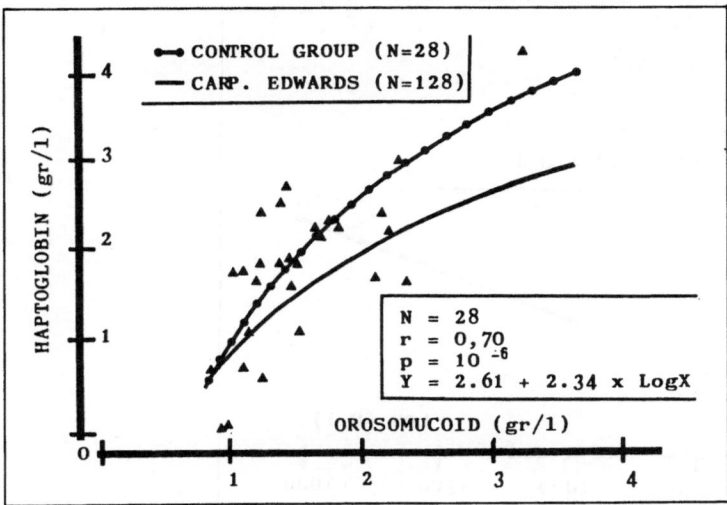

Fig. 2. Variation of haptoglobin amount in inflammation. Haptoglobin is closely correlated to orosomucoid protein (inflammation test) in the control group (dotted curve and triangles) and, at a lower level (solid curve), in the Carpentier-Edwards group.

of hemolysis. Sensitivity of hemopexin is restricted by the wide range of normal values. In all the other parameters, reticulocytes (Fig. 4), bilirubin (Fig. 5) and red cells count (Fig. 6), a nearly linear relationship with LDH can be demonstrated. However, the wide range of normal values only enables an evaluation of clinically significant hemolysis.

Influence of prosthetic valve function and site of implantation on hemolysis

Isolated aortic valve replacement was performed in 361 patients with different valve implants (Table 3). The haptoglobin and LDH values are shown in Table 4 (mean ± SEM)

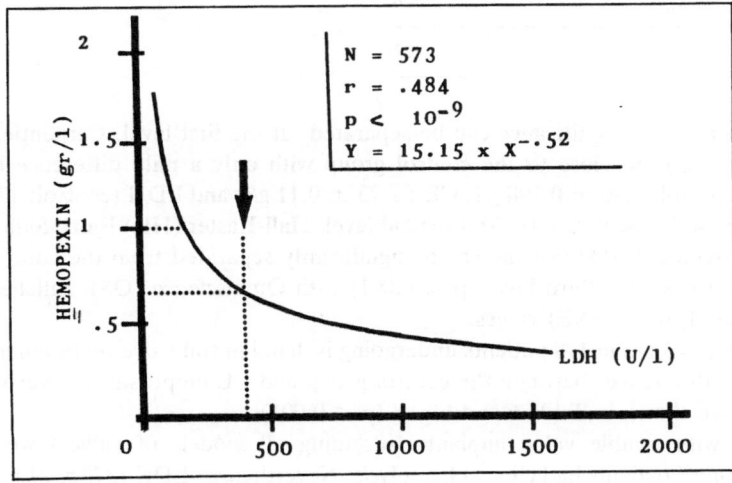

Fig. 3. Correlation curve between hemopexin and LDH.

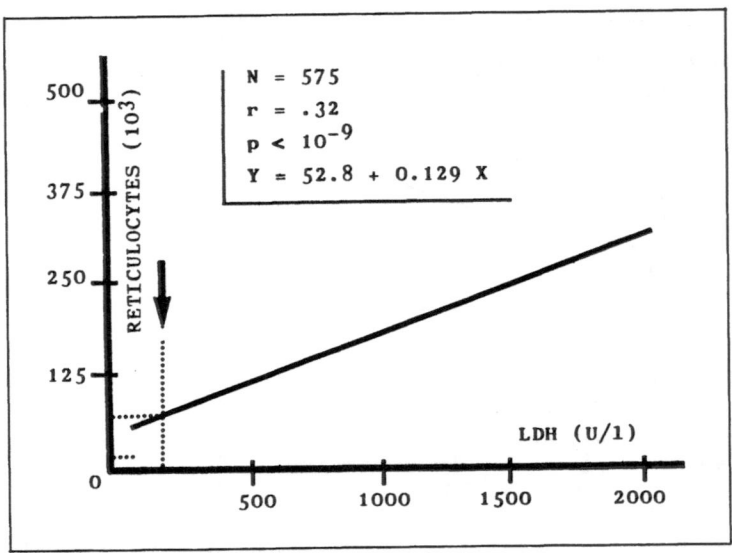

Fig. 4. Linear correlation between reticulocytes and LDH. Reticulocyte count is given in the actual amount and not as a percentage.

Table 3. Details of prosthetic valve types in isolated aortic valve replacement

Starr-Edwards	14
Lillehei-Kaster	115
Björk-Shiley	31
St. Jude Medical	26
Hall-Kaster	23
Omniscience	49
Carpentier-Edwards	95
Miscellaneous	8
	361

and in Fig. 7. Three levels of significance can be separated: at the first level, Carpentier-Edwards xenografts (CE) are close to the control group with only a mild difference in haptoglobin levels (control: 1.86 ± 0.198 g/l; CE : 1.73 ± 0.11 g/l) and LDH (control: 175 ± 5.5 u/l; CE: 198 ± 4.7; p < 0.05 u/l). At a second level, Hall-Kaster (HK) Björk-Shiley (BS) and St. Jude Medical (SJM) prostheses are significantly separated from the control group (p < 0.05) and from the third level (p < 0.001) with Omniscience (OS), Lillehei-Kaster (LK) and Starr-Edwards (SE) valves.

Hemolysis data were collected in 118 patients undergoing isolated mitral valve replacement (Table 5). Significant differences between the control group and CE bioprostheses, versus SE and SJM valves are shown in Table 6 and Fig. 8 (p < 0.001).

Thirty-two patients with double valve implants (including all models of valves) were evaluated. None of those patients had clinical hemolysis. Nevertheless, LDH (375 ± 27 u/l) and haptoglobin levels (0.047 ± 0.012 g/l) were significantly different from other groups,

Table 4. LDH levels in isolated aortic valve replacement compared to control group

Control group.	175 ± 5.5
Carpentier-Edwards . . . $P < 0.05$	198 ± 4.7
Hall-Kaster	189 ± 8.4
Björk-Shiley	211 ± 6.9
St. Jude Medical	217 ± 7.8
Omniscience . . . . $P < 0.001$	254 ± 13.5
Lillehei-Kaster	283 ± 9.4
Starr-Edwards	268 ± 11

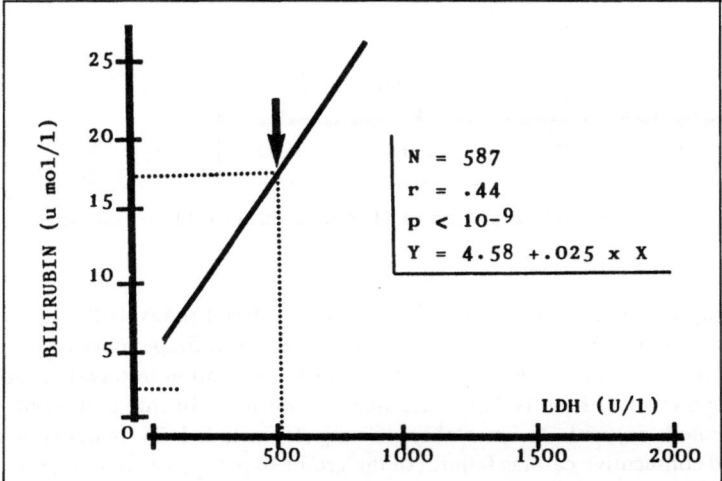

Fig. 5. Linear correlation between bilirubin and LDH. Only clinical hemolysis (LDH >500 u/l) is outside the normal bilirubin range.

Table 5. Details of prosthetic valve types in isolated mitral replacement

Carpentier-Edwards.	36
Starr-Edwards.	49
St. Jude Medical.	27
Miscellaneous	6
	118

Table 6. LDH levels in isolated mitral valve replacement compared to control group

Control group.	175 ± 5.5
Carpentier-Edwards	211 ± 13.5
Starr-Edwards . . . . . . $p < 0.001$	314 ± 12
St. Jude Medical	322 ± 40

101

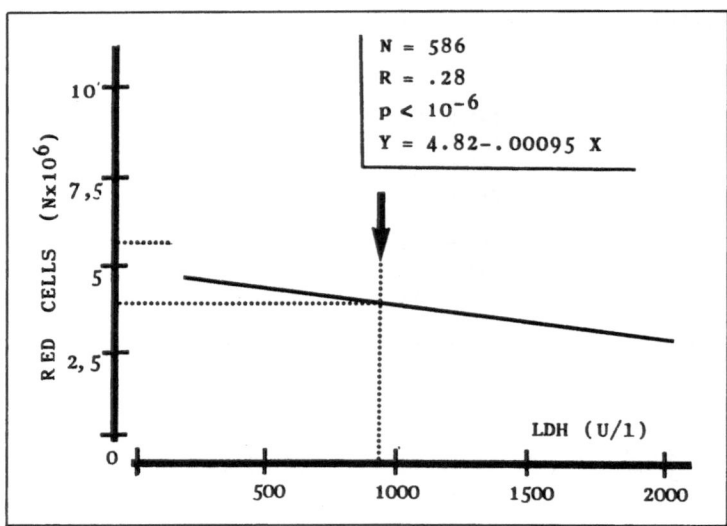

Fig. 6. Linear correlation between red cells count and LDH. Anemia in clinical hemolysis occurs at a high level of LDH.

and the level of hemolysis was the highest of all in the group without paravalvular leaks. During an 8-year period (1976–1983) paravalvular leaks occurred in 51 patients (average rate 4.1%). Forty-six patients were evaluated for hemolysis by separation into two groups. Group I included 22 patients.with an isolated insufficiency murmur. In this group only 2 patients were reoperated on with no mortality. Group II included 24 patients with paravalvular leaks and consecutive cardiac failure, of the group 18 patients were reoperated.

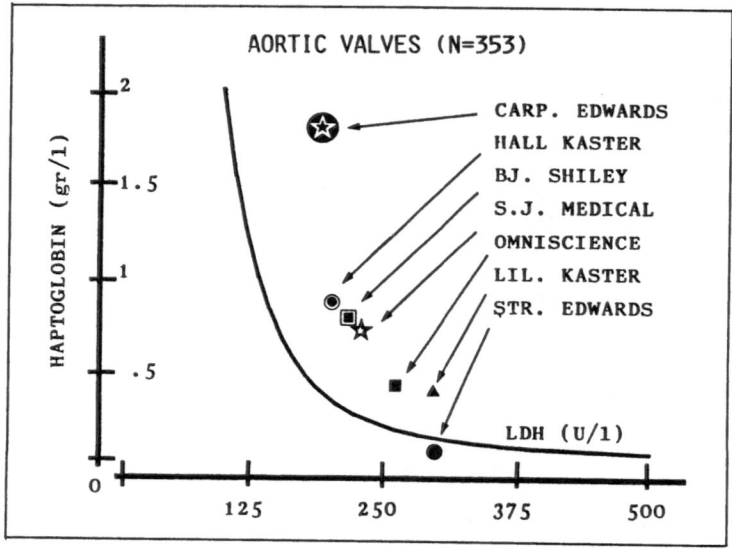

Fig. 7. Mean values of haptoglobin and LDH in isolated aortic valvular implants.

Table 7. Laboratory results and significance (p-value) between total group (PVL) compared to perivalvular leakage group I (murmur) and perivalvular leakage group II (cardiac failure)

N	PVL ⊖ 517	ⓟ	PVL ⊕ (murmur) 22	ⓟ	PVL ⊕ (card. fail.) 24
Age	58.7±.50	NS	59.1±3	NS	54.1±3
Red cells (10^6)	4.57±.02	NS	4.58±.1	10^{-9}	3.8±1
Reticulocytes (10^4)	8.45±.27	NS	8.99±1.3	10^{-9}	17.5±2
Bilirubin	11.1±.3	NS	12.4±1.2	10^{-9}	23±.5
LDH	255±4	NS	284±17	10^{-12}	729±84
Hemopexin	.90±.01	NS	.95±.93	10^{-10}	.49±0.8
Free Hb	17.5±.4	NS	20.6±2.7	NS	18.7±2
Haptoglobin	750±44	10^{-2}	161±79	10^{-4}	48±17

There was no operative mortality, but 2 patients died before reoperation, and 3 patients died later, attesting to the severity of ventricular failure.

Table 7 shows the differences between all other patients (n = 517) and those with paravalvular leaks (PVL +).

Clinical importance of evaluation of hemolysis

With the progress of cardiac valvular implants, hemolysis is no longer of clinical importance in normally functioning prostheses (1). For each type of valve individual hemolysis characteristics can be differentiated (2). Materials, orifice size, velocity of blood flow and hemodynamics certainly have a strong influence on the hemolysis level (3–5).

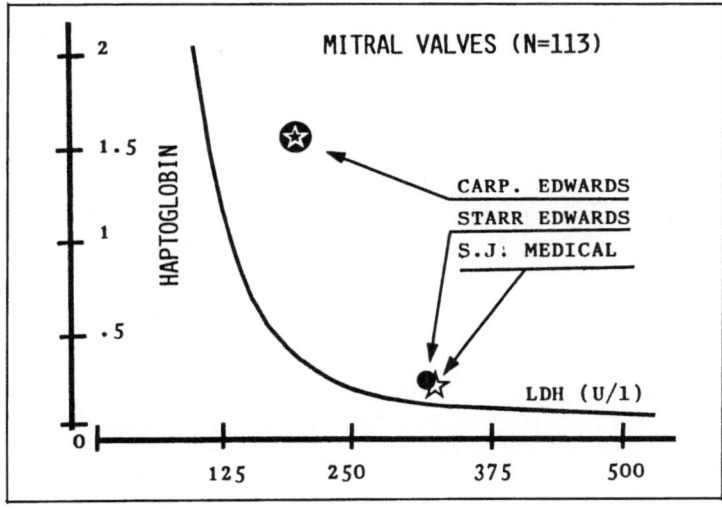

Fig. 8. Mean values of haptoglobin and LDH in isolated mitral valvular implants.

103

References

1. Horstkotte D, Haerten K, Leuner Chr. et al (1978) Chronic intravascular hemolysis following mitral valve replacement with Björk-Shiley, Lillehei-Kaster, and Starr-Edwards prostheses. Z Kardiol 67: 629
2. Horstkotte D, Aul C, Seipel L et al (1983) Influence of valve type and valve function on chronic intravascular hemolysis following mitral and aortic valve replacement using alloprostheses. Z Kardiol 72: 119
3. Crexells C, Aerichide N, Bonny Y et al (1972) Factors influencing hemolysis in valve prostheses. Am Heart J 84: 161
4. Goppel L, Küster J, Froer KL et al (1974) Das Ausmaß der intravasalen Hämolyse bei künstlichen Herzklappen unter Berücksichtigung unterschiedlicher Prothesentypen und deren Funktion. Verh Dtsch Ges Inn Med 80: 1200
5. Kastor, JA, Akbarian M, Buckley MJ et al (1968) Paravalvular leaks and hemolytic anemia following insertion of Starr-Edwards aortic and mitral valves. J Thorac Cardiovasc Surg 56:279

Authors' address:
A. Khayat, M.D.
C.H.U. Côte de Nacre
Service de Chirurgie Cardiovasculaire
14040 Caen
France

The Risk of Thromboembolism and Hemorrhage After Implantation of Heart Valve Prostheses

M. Abbate, A. Lomeo, G. Battaglia, M. Gentile, L. Carli, V. Monaca, L. Patanè, and O. Monaco

Our experience at the University of Catania, Sicily, has been to some extent similar to that in countries like South Africa, where first world technologies live close to third world social and health organizations: rheumatic disease is still endemic in Sicily; a proper anticoagulation regimen is still difficult to conduct, especially in inland areas; and patient referral from general practitioners, all the way to cardiac surgery, is still slow and often atypical.

Thromboembolic and hemorrhagic complications after heart valve replacement in Sicily

Since March 1977, when the first open-heart operation was carried out in Sicily, 781 cardiac valve replacements have been performed at our center.

The mean age of patients was low (46.6 years), and the high percentage of mitral valve replacements (64.4% MVR) and double valve replacements (17.2% DVR) shows the predominance of rheumatic disease.

When we started our work, compliance with anticoagulation was very difficult to obtain. For this reason other institutions in southern Italy chose to use biological valves only, without long-term anticoagulants. Because of the low age of our patients and considering the first disappointments with bioprostheses, we implanted a high percentage (83.3%) of mechanical valves.

We have paid what we think is a fair price in terms of significant bleeding episodes (3.5% per patient-year) but, on the other hand, our thromboembolic rate has been quite low (1.5% per patient-year). Because of these rates we looked hopefully at the possibility of using St. Jude Medical[R] valves without long-term anticoagulants.

To evaluate this possibility, we have been conducting a prospective study over the past four years, the final results of which are reported in this paper.

Heart valve replacement by St. Jude Medical prostheses with and without long-term anticoagulation

We divided all patients undergoing valve replacement into two groups according to whether they had thromboembolic risk factors (Group 2), or not (Group 1) at the time of operation (see Table 1). Group 1 patients undergoing aortic valve replacement (AVR) with St. Jude Medical[R] valves were given an antiplatelet agent only (ASA, 100 mg/day) long-term; Group 2 patients with single or double valve replacements were given long-term anticoagulants and were considered the control group. Patients in Group 1 who were put on anticoagulants for reasons other than thromboembolic episodes, and patients in Group 2 who had a mixture of cardiac prostheses were excluded from the study. Patients in Group 2 certainly carried a higher intrinsic thromboembolic risk because of preoperative NYHA class, age, pathology and hospital mortality. We thought that this protocol was suitable for judging the pure thromboembolic risk carried by any given cardiac prosthesis.

Table 1. Thromboembolic risk factors taken into consideration when classifying patients into Groups 1 and 2

Atrial fibrillation
LVF
History of thromboembolism
Coagulopathy
Thrombosis
Calcifications
Giant atrium

All patients were operated upon with the same surgical technique used by the same two
surgeons.

Results were obtained for 20 patients with AVR in Group 1 and 99 patients with single or
double valve replacements in Group 2.

Hospital mortality (first 30 days) was none in Group 1, and 6 patients (6%) in Group 2.

Follow-up was 100% in Group 1, for a period of 0.5 to 3.08 years (mean 1.59 years) for a
total of 31.8 patient-years. Follow-up of Group 2 included 94.6% of the survivors, between
0.33 and 3.91 years (mean 1.33 years) for a total of 117 patient-years. Survival probability
was 0.941 ± 0.057 for Group 1 and 0.939 ± 0.024 for Group 2 at 4 years (Figure 2).

The probability of being alive and free from major complications (reoperation, endocarditis,
bleeding, thromboembolism and leakages) was 0.423 ± 0.218 for Group 1 and $0.842 \pm$
0.084 for Group 2 ($p = 0.022$). The event-free curve is shown in Figure 3.

In Group 1 there were two reoperations for valve thrombosis at 19 and 36 months
postoperatively. One death was probably due to cerebral embolism at 12 months and a
cerebral embolism occurred at 22 months with remission.

In Group 2 there was one major bleeding episode from anticoagulation therapy, and a
myocardial infarct occurred at 22 months. The latter patient's coronary arteries were normal
preoperatively and the patient never suffered from angina, so that an embolic etiology was
suspected.

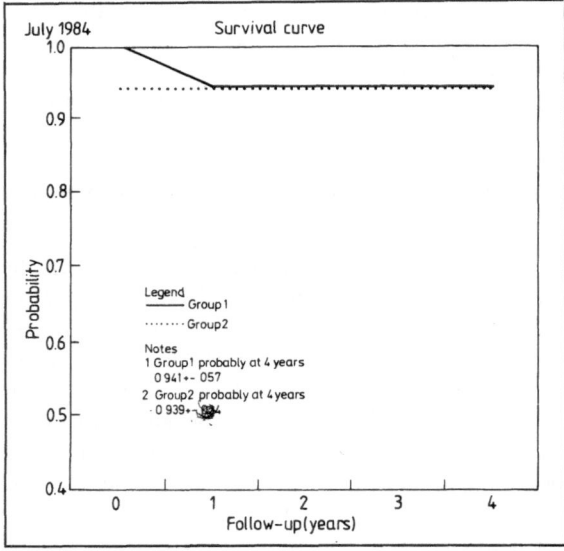

Fig. 1. Actuarial survival curve showing no significant difference between the two groups.

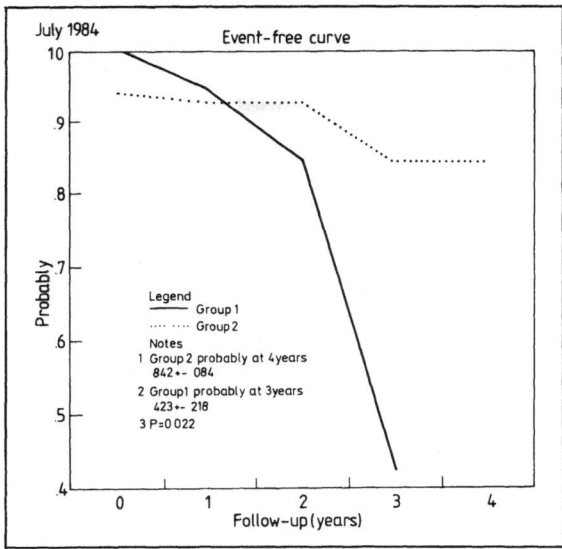

Fig. 2. Actuarial event-free curve showing a statistically significant difference between the two groups.

From our experience and that of others a low thromboembolic incidence has been demonstrated with mechanical valves associated with good anticoagulation.

In our experience the thromboembolic incidence after St. Jude Medical[R] valve replacement was 0.9% per patient-year. On the other hand, good anticoagulation may carry a reasonable hemorrhagic risk (3.5% per patient-year in our experience) which varies depending on physicians, laboratories and patients' cooperation.

We prefer mechanical valves because of the relatively low age of our patients and because Sicilian patients are reluctant to accept a second or third operation.

Our attempt to use St. Jude Medical[R] valves without anticoagulation can definitely be considered a failure. Despite a comparable survival curve, the event-free curve was much worse than that of the control group. Because of the care taken in patient selection and the high percentage of follow-up in this study, we think this regimen should not be carried out with this valve in future.

In conclusion, our current policy is to use biological valves in patients over 55 years of age and whenever anticoagulation is contraindicated; and to use mechanical valves for patients under 55 years with long-term anticoagulation. We also think biological valve patients should be anticoagulated when thromboembolic risk factors are present.

We still think a mechanical valve without anticoagulation is the ideal solution for our patient population, and we are in the process of testing a new prosthesis with the same protocol.

Authors' address:
M. Abbate, M.D.
Ospedale Vittoro Emannuele II
Via Plebiscito 628
95100 Catania
Italy

Anticoagulation and Prosthetic Heart Valves

E. Baudet

According to the Munich Terminology (1) the term prosthetic valve is synonymous with mechanical or artificial valves. Nevertheless, prosthetic valves concern not only mechanical valves but also porcine and pericardial bioprostheses (xenografts).

Although prosthetic valves have been in clinical use for more than 20 years, the ideal prosthesis which can combine durability, non thrombogenicity and minimal interference with cardiac function has not yet been made. Systemic thromboembolism remains the major cause of late mortality and morbidity. It was early recognized, when the Starr-Edwards valve was first introduced in 1961, that bare plastic and metal surfaces, as well as the cloth-covered sewing ring, predisposed to thrombus formation and thromboembolic phenomena requiring long-term anticoagulation with its own morbidity and mortality.

Thus bioprostheses have been developed to reduce the incidence of these complications. At the same time, and especially in the past 10 years, remarkable progress has been made in the designs and materials of mechanical valves. But thromboembolism remains a major time-related problem despite the use of oral anticoagulation (2), especially in patients with mechanical valves. However, long-term anticoagulation after prosthetic heart valve replacement remains a controversial question.

So, after analyzing thromboembolic factors and the incidence of thromboembolism with and without anticoagulants, we intend to answer, according to our experience, the three following questions:

What should be the early anticoagulant management after valve replacement?

Is there an optimum therapeutic level for long-term anticoagulation?

Which patients, if any, with mechanical valves could be exempt from long-term oral anticoagulation?

Terminology concerning thromboembolic phenomena

There is often some confusion in reports about thromboembolism, that include prosthetic valve thrombosis, but often without emboli as well as cerebral or peripheral emboli secondary to platelet deposition and thrombus formation on the struts and base-plate and on cloth-covered sewing rings, without interference to valve function.

It thus seems very important to differentiate between valve thrombosis and thromboembolic phenomena. Valve thrombosis originates on the valve mechanism more often, but not exclusively, on a mechanical valve, and leads to valve dysfunction. In most cases, valve thrombosis is an isolated phenomenon, without emboli from the valve thrombus. Embolic phenomena are sometimes secondary to valve thrombosis, but most of the time come from the adjacent parts of the valve mechanism, such as the cloth-covered struts and Dacron® sewing rings, which are common to mechanical and bioprosthetic valves. These embolic accidents occur without evidence of associated valve dysfunction.

Parameters differentiating normal valves, diseased valves and prosthetic valves

In a patient with chronic valvular disease, platelet survival time is abnormal. The surfaces of the valve leaflets or cusps are altered and the flow through the valve is disturbed. Patients with aortic valve disease do not usually exhibit thromboembolic episodes. In patients with mitral valve disease, and chronic atrial fibrillation and/or a large left atrium, the propensity for thrombi is due to low cardiac output and stasis of blood in the left atrium and atrial appendage. Left atrial thrombi may cause secondary emboli.

After insertion of a prosthetic valve, many other factors may contribute to thromboembolism: platelet survival, biocompatibility of valve materials, flow, valve orientation and flow velocity. Biological factors shorten platelet survival in mechanical valves (3) (5.5 ± 0.6 days versus 9.5 ± 0.2 days), while platelet kinetics are normal in bioprostheses. Also subclinical hemolysis and, in the early postoperative period, an increase of the plasma fibrinogen level (4,5) may interfere with flow properties and indicate a prethrombotic state.

The leaflet surface of a bioprosthesis seems to be non thrombogenic, but immediately after implantation the surface of the leaflets is covered by a protein layer followed by loosely attached platelets. Microthrombi appear very early on the surface of the valve, and during the first 3 or 6 weeks when they reach their maximum, anticoagulation is indicated. Despite the supposed non thrombogenicity or hemocompatibility of pyrolytic carbon, tilting disc and bileaflet valves are thrombogenic without anticoagulants, proving that factors other than the materials used cause thrombus. Obviously, the plastic and metal surfaces of ball valves are also thrombogenic. The Dacron® sewing ring and the cloth-covered seat and struts may be quite thrombogenic until they are covered by tissue. During this early phase, all these structures are not yet completely endothelialized and a fibrin apposition is possible, accounting for early embolic episodes in the first 4 postoperative months.

Flow through a prosthetic valve is a very important factor. Only unstented homografts may have a nearly central laminar flow. Most mechanical valves induce inflow and outflow disturbances because the flow is either lateral (due to the central occluder) or laminar but oblique (in tilting disc prostheses) or laminar but only in the external areas of bileaflet valves. According to valve design, velocity profiles vary depending on the major and minor flow areas, creating areas of stagnation and turbulence which are responsible for thrombus formation. Another factor that may induce turbulence, even in prostheses with central laminar flow, is the gradient across the valve, especially in the smaller sizes. Orientation of the valve, mainly for tilting disc and bileaflet prostheses, has also to be considered carefully in order to reduce the areas of stagnation, turbulence and the risk of thrombus formation. Flow velocity can also contribute to thromboembolism, especially atrial risk factors such as atrial fibrillation, intra-atrial clot responsible or not for prior embolism and increased left atrial size. The maintenance of sinus rhythm reduces the incidence of these complications after mitral valve replacement.

Incidence of thromboembolism with and without anticoagulants

Thromboembolic episodes (TE) may occur as an early or late complication of prosthetic valve replacement. Early accidents, mainly emboli without valve dysfunction, have more or less the same incidence for bioprostheses or mechanical valves (1,6). They occur mainly during the first 4 months postoperatively and are due, according to general opinion, to the fact that the cloth-covered sewing ring and implantation are thrombogenic until they are

Table 1. Incidence of valve thrombosis (VT) and systemic emboli (SE) with and without anticoagulants in patients with St. Jude Medical® prosthesis

	AVR with	AVR without	MVR with	MVR without	DVR with	DVR without
No. patients	471	65	95	10	64	3
Years per patient	2.5	1	2.3	1.8	2.1	0.36
Patient-years	1,210	65	224	18	137	1.1
No. of VT	0	4	0	1	0	1
VT % per patient-year	0	6.15	0	5.55	0	91
	└─p<0.00001─┘		└─p<0.17─┘		└─p<0.03─┘	
No. of SE	4	4	1	3	0	0
SE % per patient-year	0.33	6.15	0.44	16.66	0	0
	└─p<0.01─┘		└─p<0.001─┘		└─ N. S. ─┘	

AVR = aortic valve replacement
MVR = mitral valve replacement
DVR = double (aortic and mitral) valve replacement

endothelialized, which may take several months. Late events have a quite different rate of occurrence depending on whether the patients are on long-term anticoagulation or not. Limet et al. (7) reported TE rates for patients with Starr-Edwards valves as: 8.9% of patients receiving anticoagulants, 26.8% of patients *not* anticoagulated, and 19% of patients discontinuing anticoagulation. Data on patients receiving Björk-Shiley® valves reported by St. John Sutton et al. (8), showed that despite antiplatelet agents, thromboembolic complications were significantly more frequent in the non anticoagulated group (22%) than in the group with warfarin (7%). Table 1 shows significantly higher TE rates (both valve thromboses and systemic emboli) for patients with St. Jude Medical® valves who were not anticoagulated when compared with patients who were anticoagulated (9).

In a review of thromboembolic complications of current cardiac valvular prostheses in 1982, Edmunds (10) showed the incidence of thromboemboli was less than 2 per 100 patient-years for aortic bioprostheses without anticoagulants and for the best mechanical valves with long-term anticoagulation. After mitral valve replacement, the incidence was 4 per 100 patient-years for bioprostheses both with and without anticoagulants (since 40% to 60% of patients are anticoagulated for associated atrial risk factors) and for the best mechanical valves with long-term anticoagulants.

Early anticoagulation therapy

A higher incidence of valve thrombosis or embolic incidents has been reported for bioprostheses and mechanical valves during the first postoperative weeks. They may start in the first postoperative hours. Therefore, in 1978 we defined a protocol for early anticoagulation therapy (11) involving three steps (Table 2). Step 1: Heparin intermittent intravenous injection is started from the 6th postoperative hour, and the amount of heparin (mg/kg) is calculated according to whole blood coagulation time, the thromboembolic risk (Table 3) and patient body weight.

Step 2: Subcutaneous calcium heparin is started at the 24th postoperative hour, with an initial dose according to patient body weight, thromboembolic risk (Table 4) and secondary

Table 2. Early anticoagulant therapy after valve replacement (3 steps)

Postoperative hour	Therapy
6th	Heparin by intermittent intravenous injection
24th	Subcutaneous calcium heparin
48th	Antivitamin K
	±
	Subcutaneous calcium heparin
	±
	Nonsteroid anti-inflammatory drugs

Table 3. Early thromboembolic (TE) risk after valve surgery

High risk		Standard risk
Mitral valve replacement		Aortic valve replacement
	← Low cardiac output →	
Left atrial enlargement		
	← Atrial fibrillation →	
Previous TE episodes		Mitral conservative surgery

Table 4. Initial dosage of subcutaneous calcium heparin according to patient body weight and thromboembolic risk

Weight (kg)	Calcium heparin dose (ml) 1 mL = 25,000 IU	
	High risk	Standard risk
10	0.04	0.01
15	0.07	0.02
20	0.10	0.05
25	0.12	0.07
30	0.15	0.10
35	0.17	0.12
40	0.20	0,15
45	0.22	0.17
50	0.25	0.20
55	0.27	0.22
60	0.30	0.25
65	0.32	0.27
70	0.35	0.30
75	0.37	0.32
80	0.40	0.35
85	0.42	0.37
90	0.45	0.40
95	0.47	0.42
100	0.50	0.45

adjustment according to Howell time, in order that the patient's coagulation time should be 1.5 to 2.0 the control time.

Step 3: Oral anticoagulation is started from the 48th postoperative hour, while subcutaneous calcium heparin is simultaneously maintained until the prothrombin time (PT or Quick time) is between 25% and 35% of control values, the activated partial thromboplastin time (APPT) is 1.5 control time and the plasma fibrinogen level is normal ($<$ 4 g/l).

Control of PT, APPT and fibrinogen is done every 2 days and special attention is given to fibrinogen levels that are rapidly increasing up to 6, 10 or 11 g/l after surgery, as shown by Chakrabarti (4), with a relationship between plasma fibrinogen level and incidence of thromboemboli (3,5).

In fact, in a high velocity system, fibrinogen has no thrombogenic effect, but its role is well known in the microcirculation, such as in vascular areas with low velocity and stagnant flow areas behind prosthetic valves. A high plasma fibrinogen level influences flow properties of erythrocytes suspensions (12) and increases blood viscosity, contributing to development of thrombi. So the usual postoperative inflammatory reaction assessed by increase of the plasma fibrinogen level, in our opinion, must be considered for treatment using non-steroid anti-inflammatory drugs (Table 5).

Since this protocol was initiated in the 2,884 patients undergoing prosthetic valve replacements in both departments of cardiac surgery of the Hospital Cardiologique at Bordeaux, we have never observed an early (within 2 months) valve thrombosis or thromboembolism. This early anticoagulation therapy had no incidence of bleeding or reoperation for bleeding, and the additional anti-inflammatory drugs did not induce gastrointestinal hemorrhages. But all patients are systematically given cimetidine, starting from the first postoperative hour, to prevent stomach ulcerative lesions due to stress.

What is the optimum therapeutic level of long-term anticoagulation?

To answer this controversial question, we must consider three levels of thromboembolic risks.

Patients at *high risk* have mitral mechanical valves or mitral bioprostheses with atrial fibrillation and/or have other atrial risk factors. For these patients, well-controlled anticoagulation with antivitamin K is the most important factor in reducing the incidence of valve-related thromboembolism. Also, prothrombin time has to be maintained between 25% and 30%.

Table 5. Relationship between anticoagulant therapy and fibrinogen level

Fibrinogen $\leq$ 4 g/l:
      Subcutaneous calcium heparin stopped as soon as:
            25% $<$ PT $<$ 35% $\Big\}$ on antivitamin K
            APTT $\geq$ 1.5 control time anticoagulation

Fibrinogen $>$ 4 g/l:
      Antivitamin K
      +
      Subcutaneous calcium heparin maintained
      +
      Nonsteroid anti-inflammatory drugs
      (diclofenac, ibuprofen or indomethacin)

Patients at *standard risk* have aortic mechanical valves and mitral bioprostheses and are in sinus rhythm. If the valve size is large enough not to induce turbulences, the upper limit of prothrombin time may be extended to 40%. For patients with bioprostheses in the mitral position and in sinus rhythm, with good cardiac output, it is possible, after the first 6 postoperative months, to progressively discontinue and stop long-term anticoagulation. In this case, antivitamin K has to be replaced by antiplatelet agents (low doses of aspirin eventually combined with dipyridamole). Also, the fibrinogen level and coagulation have to be checked at regular intervals to detect any secondary and temporary hypercoagulability. Patients at *low risk* have aortic bioprostheses and aortic mechanical valves, and if a mechanical valve is present, it is not restrictive and there is a well preserved cardiac function. In patients with aortic bioprostheses, anticoagulation may be discontinued 3 months postoperatively with or without antiplatelet agents. In patients with mechanical valves, risk depends on the type of valve (lateral flow, central flow, laminar flow) and its orientation. The prothrombin time in these patients should be between 30% and 40%. For some, discontinuing anticoagulation may be considered, in special circumstances.

Is oral anticoagulation necessary for all patients with mechanical valves?

Long-term oral anticoagulants should be given permanently to all patients with mechanical valves except in certain circumstances. The following parameters should be checked when considering no anticoagulants:
- Bleeding complications associated with long-term anticoagulation increase with age over 70 years as well as in children exposed to the trauma of active life.
- Only valves in the aortic position should be considered for no oral anticoagulation maintenance.
- The hemodynamics of the valve should be optimal. Bileaflet prostheses, despite the fact that they do not meet the criteria of an ideal prosthesis, are at present, in our opinion, the best mechanical valves in terms of hemodynamic performance.
- Left ventricular function is a major factor in providing good cardiac output and high flow velocity.
- Initial temporary anticoagulation should be maintained with subcutaneous administration of heparin to prevent rebound phenomena and hypercoagulability when oral anticoagulation is discontinued.
- The fibrinogen level and coagulation should be controlled at regular intervals to be sure that there is isocoagulability.
- Antiplatelet agents should be given systematically.
- Since the use of bioprostheses is contraindicated in children, aortic mechanical valves in this special group of patients are the most likely to be not anticoagulated long-term. In the elderly, bioprostheses should be used, except in cases of a small aortic annulus. In these patients, the risk of anticoagulation or no anticoagulation has to be analyzed in the same way as mentioned above.

Anticoagulation in patients with prosthetic heart valves

Anticoagulation is indicated for all patients with prosthetic heart valves and should be given permanently to all patients with mechanical valves (with some exceptions in the aortic position) and to patients with mitral bioprostheses when atrial risk factors or atrial fibrillation are present.

The plasma fibrinogen level has to be considered mainly in the early postoperative period, but its levels should be systematically measured in the late and periodical coagulation controls because its increase, due to many causes (e.g. dental infection, tonsillitis) may account for secondary prothrombin time maladjustment in which nonsteroid anti-inflammatory drugs should be prescribed at the same time that the dose of antivitamin K is adjusted.

Durability being equal, the ideal bioprosthetic or mechanical valve should be not require long-term anticoagulation. Up to now, the necessary oral anticoagulation proves that despite supposedly bio- or hemocompatibility, the material used for mechanical valves remains more or less thrombogenic. The hemodynamics of prosthetic valves, despite their recent and remarkable progress, especially in small diameters, has to be improved. Turbulences existing in ball and tilting disc valves have been reduced in the new generation of bileaflet prostheses, but their fixed structures in the orifice (struts or hinges) remain potential thrombogenic areas.

References

1. Sebening F, Klövekorn WP, Meisner H et al (eds) (1979) Bioprosthetic Cardiac Valves: Proceedings of the First International Symposium on Tissue Heart Valves. Munich, April 5–7. Deutsches Herzzentrum München
2. Chesebro JM, Fuster.V, Elveback LR et al (1983) Trial of combined warfarin plus dipyridamole or aspirin therapy in prosthetic heart valve replacement: Danger of aspirin compared with dipyridamole. Am J Cardiol 51: 1537
3. Avellaneda A (1983) Les accidents thrombo-emboliques et neuropsychiatriques et leur incidence à court et long terme chez les porteurs de prothèses valvulaires cardiaques. Thèse de Doctorat en Médécine, n° 143, Bordeaux
4. Chakrabarti R, Hocking ED, Fearnley GR (1976) Reaction pattern to three stresses: electroplexy, surgery and myocardial infarction of fibrinolysis and plasma fibrinogen. J Clin Pathol 22: 659–662
5. Fulton RM, Duckett, K (1976) Plasma fibrinogen and thromboemboli after myocardial infarction. Lancet 2: 1161
6. Cohn LH, Gallucci V (1982) Cardiac Bioprostheses: Proceedings of the Second International Symposium on Tissue Heart Valves. Rome, May 17–19. Yorke Medical Books, New York
7. Limet R, Lepage G, Grondin CM (1977) Thromboembolic complications with the cloth-covered Starr-Edwards aortic prosthesis in patients not receiving anticoagulants. Ann Thorc Surg 23: 529
8. St John Sutton MG, Miller GAH, Oldershaw PJ et al (1978) Anticoagulants and the Björk-Shiley prosthesis. Experience of 390 patients. Br Heart J 40: 558
9. Baudet EM, Oca CC, Roques FX et al (1984) Five and half year's experience with the St. Jude Medical cardiac valve prosthesis: Early and late results of 737 valve replacements in 671 patients. Fourth International Symposium on the St. Jude Medical Valve, Montego Bay, Jamaica, March 12–14 (in press)
10. Edmunds LH Jr (1982) Thromboembolic complications of current cardiac valvular prostheses. Ann Thorac Surg 34: 96
11. Baudet EM (1983) Management of early anticoagulant therapy after valve replacement. Simposio Internationale sulle Malattie Valvolari Cardiache Acquisite, Acireale – Catania (Sicily), June 20–23. Acta Mediterranea (in press)
12. Wells RE, Gawronski TH, Cox PJ et al (1964) Influence of fibrinogen on flow properties of erythrocytes suspensions. Am J Physiol 207: 1035

Author's address:
E. M. Baudet, M.D.
Dept. of Cardiovascular Surgery
Hopital Cardiologique
Ave de Magellan
33604 Bordeaux
France

Valve Malfunction and Heart Valve Replacement in Patients at Risk

D. Horstkotte and F. Loogen

Since its early beginnings prosthetic heart valve replacement has been related to some specific problems, the importance of which has changed in the last decades, but which continue to be matters for discussion. First, this includes a consequent diagnosis of prosthetic valve malfunctions, made in time to initiate an early therapy. Frequently, this therapy consists in surgical revision of the malfunctioning prosthesis; sometimes reoperation can be avoided by early induction of conservative therapy (prosthetic valve endocarditis, prosthetic valve thrombosis). Regarding prosthetic valve malfunctions, paraprosthetic leakages and dysfunctions of the valve occluder itself which may be caused by infective endocarditis, prosthetic valve thrombosis, tissue ingrowth, material defects or a degeneration of the biological valve material must be differentiated. A variety of case reports document the importance of diagnostics in due time and immediate initiation of an adequate therapy for the successful management of prosthetic valve malfunctions (1,2). Normally noninvasive examinations before initiating adequate therapeutic measures are sufficient to achieve an accurate diagnosis of a prosthesis malfunction (cf. chapter 7.2).

Secondly, the demands made of diagnostics and indications for prosthetic valve replacement are of a special kind for patients where the lesion has to be operated upon under certain circumstances. This is the case if valve replacement has to be performed in patients with severe right and/or left ventricular impairment, in young, or old patients.

Additionally, the decision to operate and the performance of the operation itself in cases of acute infective endocarditis of native valves or in prosthetic valve endocarditis requires special considerations (3–5). Finally, special therapeutic measures are also necessary for patients with heart valve replacement in cases of pregnancy (6).

Myocardial dysfunction implicates special requirements for judging the indications for prosthetic heart valve replacement if this impairment is equivalent to valve failure or even worse, and its cause cannot be explained by the valve failure alone. In these cases postoperative improvement of left ventricular impairment and, therefore, the physical capacity lag behind the result usually expected after valve implantation. Valve replacement is allied with an increased operative risk in these cases. For mitral stenoses or medium degree combined mitral valve lesions and advanced left ventricular impairment, a marked improvement of the clinicial classification by operation is unattainable in most cases.

Because of the very poor prognosis of severe valvular aortic stenosis and valve lesions with a severe left ventricular volume overload (7), however, there is no alternative to prosthetic heart valve replacement even if a severe left ventricular impairment exists (7–9). Additionally, for severe mitral and/or aortic valve incompetence and severe aortic stenosis, preoperatively it cannot be definitely distinguished how far an impairment of left ventricular pump function must be regarded as a consequence of the pressure or volume load. Furthermore, the exact point at which cardiac dysfunction is associated with irreversible tissue damage cannot be determined (10). In mild or moderate aortic valve lesions, however, a significant improvement of impaired left ventricular function cannot necessarily be expected, because in these patients one would not expect heart failure to be related predominantly to the aortic lesion (8).

When it is difficult to decide whether a myocardial dysfunction was originally related to a valve failure or if there is an additional myocardial component, patient history, and if available, the clinical follow-up, may provide further information. In cases of doubt, which have in general to be considered as very rare, histological examinations of tissue from endomyocardial catheter biopsies may clarify the situation.

For prosthetic valve replacement in infancy and adolescence hemodynamic properties must be particularly considered. As very frequently only smaller protheses can be implanted without producing prosthesis dysfunctions or interference with the ventricular geometrics, with the increase in cardiac output related to growth, a re-operation is frequently indispensable (11) if the physical capacity becomes limited again. Prior to such an operation, a catheterization at rest and under ergometer exercise with measurements of the pulmonary artery pressure, the left ventricular end-diastolic pressure, and the transprosthetic gradient at the mitral- or aortic valve must always be carried out to objectify an exercise-induced obstruction of the blood flow through the prosthesis. In infancy, in cases with an absolute indication for operation, a valve-conserving procedure should be chosen. With only a relative indication for valve replacement in infancy, an operation should be postponed until it is possible to implant valve sizes which will also provide satisfactory hemodynamic results when the cardiac output increases. With the deferment of the first manifestation of symptoms of heart valve disease to older age (12), the questions of preoperative exclusion and the detection of concomitant coronary artery and peripheral arterial occlusive diseases gain in importance.

Because of the very poor prognosis of severe aortic valve failures and mitral incompetences, a higher age itself does not mean a contraindication for valve operation in cases of these lesions (7). Preoperative coronary angiography together with an invasive study of the hemodynamic severity of the valve failure should be routinely performed for male patients over 40 years old, and for female patients above 45 years of age, even if there are no symptoms of coronary artery disease (13). Because the risk of operation for valve replacement and concomitant coronary revascularization is not higher than that of isolated prosthetic valve implantation, according to the higher benefit for the patient regarding freedom from symptoms and long-term prognosis, the simultaneous revascularization of all coronary arteries with significant stenoses during heart surgery is recommended (13, 14). Doppler echocardiography for the detection of hemodynamically relevant stenoses of cerebral arteries before valve replacement in older patients is also indispensable. With a mean incidence of clinically manifest stenoses and cerebral artery occlusions in patients aged 65 and above of 0.5% yearly (15), we have to expect hemodynamically relevant stenoses of the supra-aortic arteries in more than 5% of the 65-year-old patients, and in more than 8% of the 70-year-old patients. Hemodynamically relevant stenoses require a correction, which normally has to be performed prior to the heart valve replacement, since under the conditions of extracorporal circulation, stenoses which are at first compensated, may decompensate and cause ischaemic damage.

The indications for surgical intervention in infective endocarditis of native as well as of prosthetic heart valves are still a matter of controversial discussion, even though many centres recently recommended early surgical intervention (5, 11, 16).

118

On the one hand, the implantation of prosthetic material into infected tissue contradicts basic surgical principles. Very frequently the price of repeated operations has to be paid, so that – if possible – a conservative treatment of the infected area should be aspired to. On the other hand, very frequently, an emergency operation is inevitable because of progressive valve dysfunction with concomitant volume load and myocardial damage, as well as complications in terms of persistent sepsis despite antibiotic therapy, septic embolisms or acute renal failure. If the course of native valve endocarditis, and particularly prosthetic valve endocarditis, is accompanied by one of these complications, we regard an emergency operation to be indicated (16). In cases of conservatively compensated left heart failure, operation should be recommended if there is an isolated infection of the aortic valve or of both left-sided heart valves, while in the case of isolated mitral valve involvement conservative treatment can be continued. Vegetations documented by echocardiography, especially when increasing in size (17–19), and endocarditis caused by staphylococci, enterococci and gram-negative germs (20), give additional arguments for an immediate surgical intervention. Endocarditis caused by staphylococci or gram-negative germs can very seldom be treated conservatively, fungal endocarditis almost never (20).

Pregnancy poses a special problem for patients after heart valve replacement with mechanical prostheses, because anticoagulation with derivatives of cumarin (Marcumar®, Warfarin®, Sintrom®) able to pass the placenta can – at least in the first trimenon – act teratogenously (21, 22). Therefore in this case an anticoagulation with heparin derivatives, not penetrating the placenta, is necessary. Besides the cumarin-induced embriopathies a high rate of abortus and of bleeding complications must be expected (6), especially for the fetus. For these reasons for women expecting pregnancy, a biological valve replacement has to be taken into consideration after comprehensive discussion of the necessity of a subsequent reoperation, and the risks accompanying it.

References

1. Ansbro J, Clark R, Gerbode F (1978) Successful surgical correction of an embolized prosthetic valve poppet. J Thorac Cardiovasc Surg 72:130
2. Horstkotte D, Körfer R (1983) Prosthetic valve endocarditis with embolization of a Smeloff-Cutter aortic valve prosthesis: Diagnosis, operative management, and clinical and hemodynamic findings up to 3 years postoperatively. Z Kardiol 72:476
3. Bircks W, Reidemeister Ch, Sadony V et al (1972) Diagnostic and therapeutic problems of septicemia after valvular replacement. J Cardiovasc Surg 13:385
4. Dismukes WE (1981) Prosthetic valve endocarditis: Factors influencing outcome and recommendations for therapy. In: Bisno AL (ed) Treatment of Infective Endocarditis. Grune and Stratton, New York, p 167
5. Stulz P, Pfisterer M, Hasse J et al (1984) Die Prothesendokarditis – eine chirurgische Indikation! Schweiz med Wschr 114:1586
6. Hall JG, Pauli RM, Wilson KM (1980) Maternal and fetal sequelae of anticoagulation during pregnancy. Am J Med 68:122
7. Horstkotte D, Loogen F, Kleikamp G et al (1983) The influence of heart-valve replacement on the natural history of isolated mitral, aortic, and multivalvular disease: Clinical results in 783 patients up to 8 years after implantation of Björk-Shiley tilting-disc prostheses. Z Kardiol 72:494
8. Smith N, McAnulty JH, Rahimtoola SH (1978) Severe aortic stenosis with impaired left ventricular function and clinical heart failure: Results of valve replacement. Circulation 58:255
9. Schwarz F, Flameng W, Thormann J et al (1978) Recovery from myocardial failure after aortic valve replacement. J Thorac Cardiovasc Surg 75:854
10. McGoon DC (1976) Valvular replacement and ventricular function. J Thorac Cardiovasc Surg 72:326

11. Horstkotte D (1985) Indikationen und diagnostische Maßnahmen für Zweiteingriffe nach Herzklappenersatz. J Thorac Cardiovasc Surg 33:12
12. Loogen F, Horstkotte D (1982) Therapy of valvular heart disease. In: Bleifeld W, Mathey D (eds) Therapy of Cardiovascular Disease. Thieme, Stuttgart – New York, p 21
13. Körfer R, Bircks W, Horstkotte D et al (1983) Cardiac valve replacement and simultaneous myocardial revascularization. Z Kardiol 72:18
14. Kirklin JW, Kouchoukos NT (1981) Aortic valve replacement without myocardial revascularisation (Editorial). Circulation 63:252
15. Kannel WB (1976) Some lessons in cardiovascular epidemiology from Framingham. Am J Cardiol 37:269
16. Horstkotte D, Körfer R, Loogen F et al (1984) Prosthetic valve endocarditis: Clinical findings and management. Eur Heart J 5 (Suppl C): 117
17. Schelbert HR, Müller OF (1972) Detection of fungal vegetations involving a Starr-Edwards mitral prosthesis by means of ultrasound. Vasc Surg 6:20
18. Srivastava TN, Hussain M, Gray LA et al (1976) Echocardiographic diagnosis of a stuck Björk-Shiley aortic valve prosthesis. Chest 70:94
19. Dillon T, Meyer RA, Korfhagen JC et al (1980) Management of infective endocarditis using echocardiography. J Pediatr 96:552
20. Horstkotte D, Rosin H (1984) Therapie und Prophylaxe der infektiösen Endokarditis. Schweiz med Wschr 114:1575
21. Pettifor JM, Benson R (1975) Congenital malformations associated with the administration of oral anticoagulants during pregnancy. J Pediatr 86:459
22. Shaul WL, Hall JG (1977) Multiple congenital anomalies associated with oral anticoagulants. Am J Obstet Gynecol 127:191

Authors' address:

Dr. Dieter Horstkotte
Medizinische Klinik der
Universität Düsseldorf
Moorenstraße 5
4000 Düsseldorf
F.R.G.

Incidence, Clinical Findings and Management of Prosthetic Valve Malfunction

R. Körfer and D. Horstkotte

The term prosthetic valve malfunction describes a situation in which the implanted device does not accomplish its function as a valvular substitute. This situation can be caused either by a periprosthetic leak or by true dysfunction of the prosthetic valve. Prosthetic valve dysfunction can be due to valve thrombosis, thrombendocarditis involving the prosthesis, mechanical disorder of the valve including wear or degeneration of xenografts, or tissue ingrowth (Table 1). Paravalvular and prosthetic dysfunction can occur separately or together, and in the individual case discerning between these two malfunctions may be difficult.

Table 1. Prosthetic valve malfunction

- Paraprosthetic leak
- Prosthetic valve dysfunction
  - Prosthetic thrombosis
  - Thrombendocarditis
  - Mechanical disorder
    (incl. wear and degeneration of tissue valves)
  - Tissue ingrowth

Clinical features of prosthetic valve malfunction

Depending on etiology and hemodynamic effects, the clinical features of a malfunctioning valve include a wide spectrum of details which are more or less dominating and present in most of the cases: new murmurs, dyspnea, hemolysis, symptoms of heart failure, symptoms of infection, peripheral embolisms, arrhythmias, angina pectores and syncopes. For example, the development of fever associated with the auscultation of a new murmur, and increasing rates of hemolysis point strongly to the presence of prosthetic valve endocarditis. Nevertheless for complete evaluation with subsequent optimal management, several noninvasive and invasive examinations may be necessary

Diagnostic tools of prosthetic valve malfunction

Auscultation and phonocardiography as much as ever lead to correct diagnoses in many cases (1, 2) while echocardiography, especially when combined with Doppler ultrasound, is another important tool for confirming the diagnosis noninvasively (3, 4). A murmur due to valvular incompetence was always present in our patients with a paravalvular leak and in 76% of patients with prosthetic valve thrombosis. A stenotic murmur was heard in more than 80% of the patients with proven tissue ingrowth, in 42% of the patients with valve

Table 2. Prosthetic valve malfunction

Diagnostic tools

- Physical examination
- Auscultation, PCG
- Pulse recording
- ECG
- Laboratory findings
- Echo (and Doppler)
- X-ray and fluoroscopy
- Gated blood pool
- Cardiac catheterization and angiography

Table 3. Auscultatory findings with prosthetic valve malfunction (n = 103)

● New murmurs of valve regurgitation	
Periprosthetic leak	100%
Prosthetic thrombosis	76%
● New stenotic murmurs	
Tissue ingrowth	82%
Prosthetic thrombosis	42%
Thrombendocarditis	21%
● Diminution or loss of prosthetic clicks	
Prosthetic thrombosis	93%
Thrombendocarditis	13%

thrombosis and in 20% of patients with infective endocarditits of the prosthesis. The loss of the opening click is an indication of valve thrombosis (Tables 2 and 3).

Paravalvular leak

The most frequent malfunction after heart valve replacement is a paravalvular leak (5), which is observed in 3 to 8% of all patients undergoing prosthetic valve replacement. In our patients the frequency was 4.1%, and in 1.8% reoperation was necessary. Usually a leak occurs within days or months postoperatively. Predisposing factors are: inflammatory or severe degenerative tissue alterations at the site of valvular attachment, or imperfect surgical management, e.g., incomplete removal of calcified tissue, inadequate number of sutures, loose sutures and improper sizing. In the mitral position the incidence of leaks has been somewhat higher than in the aortic position.

Clinical symptoms of periprosthetic leak are similar to those of valve incompetence. An indication of a large leak is abnormal tilting of the prosthesis during the cardiac cycle. A tilting movement of more than 8° in the aortic, and more than 10° (Fig. 1) in the mitral position seen during fluoroscopy or angiography is highly indicative of dehiscence of the valve (6–8). Other important signs of paravalvular leak can be found by echocardiography (9, 10). In nearly all patients we found a rocking opening of the valve occluder and a premature opening of a leaking mitral valve prosthesis due to increased left atrial pressure. In leaks of the aortic valve prostheses, a fluttering of the mitral valve and/or the interventricular septum is seen in most cases (Table 4).

122

Table 4. Echocardiographic findings with paravalvular leaks

- Rocking opening motion of valve occluder (hump) 94%
- Premature opening of mitral prostheses 88%
  (A_2-MVO)

- Diastolic fluttering of mitral valve and/or IVS 89%
  (leaking aortic prostheses)
- Signs of volume overload increasing LVEDD or LA 66%

A_2-MVO = interval between the aortic segment of the second heart sound and the opening movement of the mitral prosthesis; IVS = interventricular septum; LVEDD = end-diastolic diameter of the left ventricle; LA = diameter of the left atrium

Finally, in patients with paravalvular leaks, red cell damage is consistently more pronounced than in normally functioning prostheses. The degree of hemolysis is a reliable indicator of the functional integrity of the prosthesis (11). The increase of LDH is a simple but sufficient parameter of chronic intravascular hemolysis (12) in patients with proven leaks or other valve malfunctions in comparison to normally working prostheses (11). Only in one type of prosthesis (Lillehei-Kaster) did we find some overlapping of LDH-values in those patients

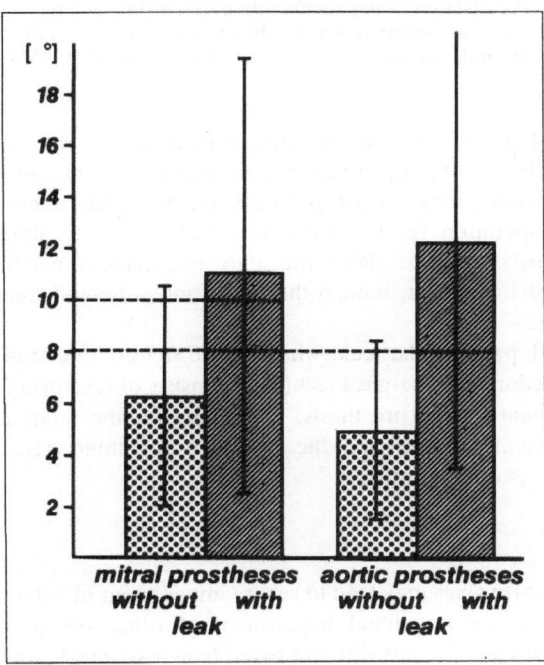

Fig. 1. Tilting movement of prosthetic valves during fluoroscopy or angiography. In mitral prostheses the tilting angle was measured to be 6 ± 4° without a perivalvular leak and 11 ± 8° in valves with proven perivalvular regurgitation. In aortic prostheses we found tilting movements of 5 ± 3° in valves without leaks and 12 ± 8° in leaking prostheses.

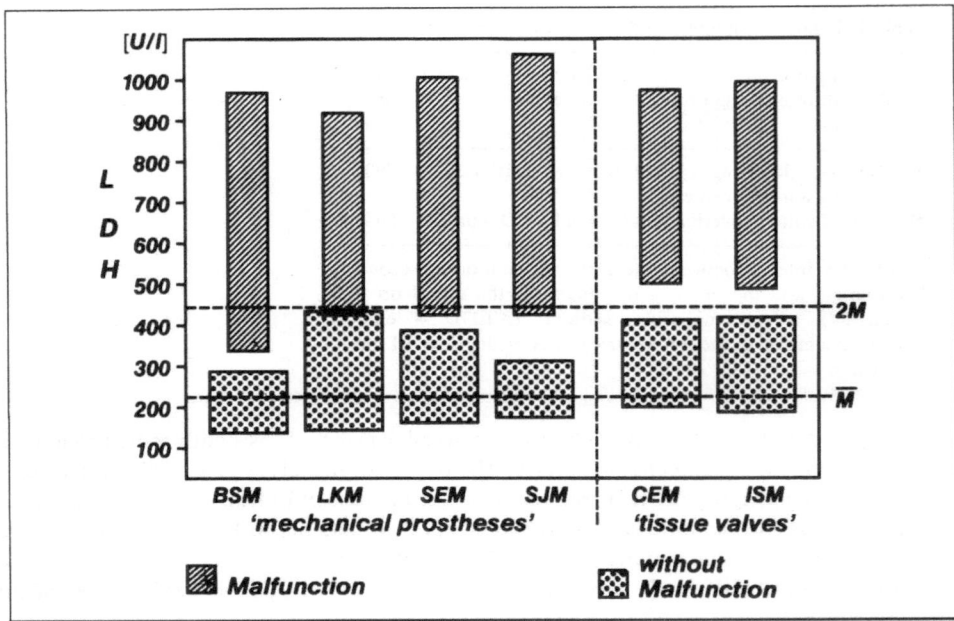

Fig. 2. Intravascular hemolysis by means of the LDH-levels in patients with normally functioning mitral valve prostheses and with proven prosthetic valve malfunction. BSM = Björk-Shiley, LKM = Lillehei-Kaster, SEM = Starr-Edwards, SJM = St. Jude Medical, CEM = Carpentier-Edwards, ISM = Ionescu-Shiley.

with and without valve malfunction (Fig. 2). However, the degree of hemolysis does not correlate with the hemodynamic significance of periprosthetic regurgitation (11). Occasionally, leaks of lesser hemodynamic importance may cause disproportionate hemolytic anemia. Consequently, the indication for reoperation for a paravalvular leak is nearly almost recurrent congestive heart failure. In our series there was only one patient needing reoperation for uncompensated hemolytic anemia, though there was only a hemodynamically mild paraprosthetic regurgitation.

The risk of reoperation in patients with paravalvular leaks who have no signs of infection is not higher than that at the initial procedure. The surgical technique consists of resuturing at the paravalvular leak or re-replacement of the prosthesis, depending on the anatomic situation the presence of additional thrombi, the design of the previously implanted valve or the quality of the tissue at the site of re-attachment.

Prosthetic valve thrombosis

Thrombi that develop on prosthetic heart valves may lead to severe impediment of valvular function. Also thrombi may cause severe functional impairment of other organs by embolization. The development of new valve designs with improved hemodynamic features and the use of new materials with less thrombogenicity has reduced the rates of thromboembolic complications (5, 13). However, the risk of valve thrombosis is a uniformly distributed risk over the lifetime of a mechanical valve. Up to now, any mechanical valve, regardless of design, position or placement, requires long-term anticoagulation. Yet anticoagulation carries its own morbidity and mortality, and it cannot absolutely prevent thromboembolism (5, 14). However, the benefits of anticoagulation exceed the hemorrhagic side effects seen with mechanical prostheses. With respect to tissue valves there has been a lower rate of thromboembolism without such a great need for anticoagulation in patients with sinus rhythm. However, xenografts have no significant advantages in patients having unstable atrial rhythms, previous thromboembolic events or unfavourable anatomy, e.g. cardiac chamber dilatations.

The diagnosis of prosthetic thrombosis can be suggested after arterial embolism. Without such an event, a thrombosis may be discovered only if the closing and/or opening mechanism is disturbed. Examinations of high diagnostic value are auscultation (Table 3), if a diminution or loss of prosthetic clicks can be found, and echocardiography (Table 5).

A rounded opening motion of the occluder is seen in more than 80%. In two-thirds of the patients a premature opening of the mitral prosthesis and a missed, incomplete, reduced, delayed, or intermittent opening motion of the occluder can be documented.

Surgical management of prosthetic valve thrombosis consists of prosthetic valve re-replacement. Cleaning of the prosthesic seems to be unfavorable because of increased thrombogenicity of the remaining surface. The risk of reoperation is low if the patient is operated upon in time, otherwise the outcome is dependent on previous damage of vital organs. Finally, it should be mentioned that in very rare cases a successful thrombolysis might be possible.

Prosthetic thrombendocarditis

Prosthetic valve endocarditis is an exceedingly serious and not uncommon complication in patients who have had prosthetic valve replacement. In most reports prosthetic valve endocarditis is subdivided into a so-called high risk group with early onset of symptoms within 2 months of operation and a so-called low risk group with late onset of symptoms. Early prosthetic valve endocarditits is usually attributable to septic complications of surgery and is characterized by infections with more virulent organisms. Late prosthetic valve endocarditis is usually caused by transient bacteremia related to dental manipulations, surgical wounds or to other sources that were not adequately covered by prophylactic antibiotic therapy.

Table 5. Echocardiographic findings with prosthetic thrombosis or tissue ingrowth (n = 19)

● Rounded opening motion of occluder (hump)	84%
● Premature opening of mitral prostheses (A_2-MVO)	68%
● Missed incomplete or reduced, delayed, intermittent } Opening motion of the occluder	63%
● Dense echos within the prosthetic valve opening area	42%

(false positive: reverberations)

125

The outcome of such infections, whether treated medically or surgically, is generally dismal, and according to recent literature, mortality rates range between 30% and 77% (15–18). The incidence of prosthetic valve endocarditis has decreased markedly in the past years with the use of prophylactic antibiotics prior to surgery, shorter operating time and improved antibiotic prophylaxis for minor operative or invasive medical interventions. In our experience over 16 years, 1.4% of patients developed early endocarditis, and 2.3% had late endocarditis within 15 years postoperatively. Infections of the aortic valve have been more frequent than those of the mitral valve (18).

The clinical features of prosthetic valve infection are for the most part the same as those that characterize infective endocarditis of native valves. The patient's deterioration is parallel with the gradual development of heart failure due to a progressive impairment of the opening or closing movement of the valve poppet by growth of bacteria, or less often by fungi. Diffuse inflammatory invasion of the anulus may lead to almost complete tearing away of the prosthesis (19). Embolization of vegetations may cause severe dysfunction in vital organs.

Treatment of prosthetic valve endocarditis is a challenging and difficult problem. The principal questions are, how long a primary trial with antibiotics should last, and whether and when a reoperation should be performed (15, 20). Since mortality rates of medically treated patients with early onset of symptoms is extremely high (up to 90%) (15) surgical replacement of the prosthesis is the most promising decision.

Nevertheless one has to bear in mind that there is no assurance that the newly implanted prosthesis will not be infected again.

In the lower risk group with late onset of symptoms of prosthetic valve endocarditis a reoperation is indicated when signs and symptoms of progressive heart failure, embolism, fungal endocarditis, persistent septicemia or renal failure are present (18).

Mechanical disorders of prosthetic heart valves

At the present time most mechanical valves used throughout the world have an excellent record of durability with low failure rates, though the recent reports of strut fractures of the Björk-Shiley Convexo-concave model have demonstrated that the question of durability may appear at any time (21). With the exception of this series, failures of mechanical valves are seen only in individual cases.

Dysfunction of caged-ball prostheses can be due to either wear of the occluder, known as ball variance (22, 23), with the possibility of sticking or embolization, or to strut fracture (24). Dysfunction of disc valves can also be produced by fracture of the occluder or the strut, which became known in an increasing number of patients with Björk-Shiley valves especially in the 29 mm size mitral prostheses (21, 25, 26, 27).

Moreover, jamming of the occluder may be caused by chordae tendineae between disc and rim, overhanging knots, long sutures and catheters for postoperative monitoring. In most instances mechanical failure of a prosthesis is a disastrous complication and survival is rare.

Failure of tissue valves due to wear, degenerations or calcification is a well-known problem (28–30). The life of a tissue valve is influenced by the kind of tissue, sterilization methods, preservation modalities, mounting techniques, patient age and additional diseases.

Although there is an acceleration in the rate of valve failures after 5 years, the incidence of late failures remains under study. Occasionally breakdown of a tissue valve can be seen immediately (bleeding into a leaflet) or a short time after operation (leaflet disruption),

Table 6. Frequency of reoperation*

	MVR		AVR		DVR	
	BSM (n=442)	SJM (n=167)	BSA (n=393)	SJA (n = 147)	BSM+BSA (n=105)	SJM+SJA (n=64)
Mean follow-up (months)	36.4±18.4	23.2±10.3	39.3±18.6	22.2±9.4	39.8±21.6	21.4±10.7
Valve thrombosis	3		3			
Prosthetic valve endocarditis	1		4		1	
Paravalvular leakage	11	2	9	3	3	1
Mechanical failure	1					
Σ	16	2	16	3	4	1
Reop./100 patient-years	1.19	0.62	1.24	1.10	1.15	0.88

* Due to valve thrombosis, infectious prosthetic valve endocarditis, paravalvular leakage, or mechanical failure.

resulting in severe hemodynamic compromise. Prompt valve replacement is mandatory in these cases. Management of mechanical disorders of prosthetic cardiac valves can be elective in cases with slowly increasing dysfunction which is mostly seen in xenografts or as an

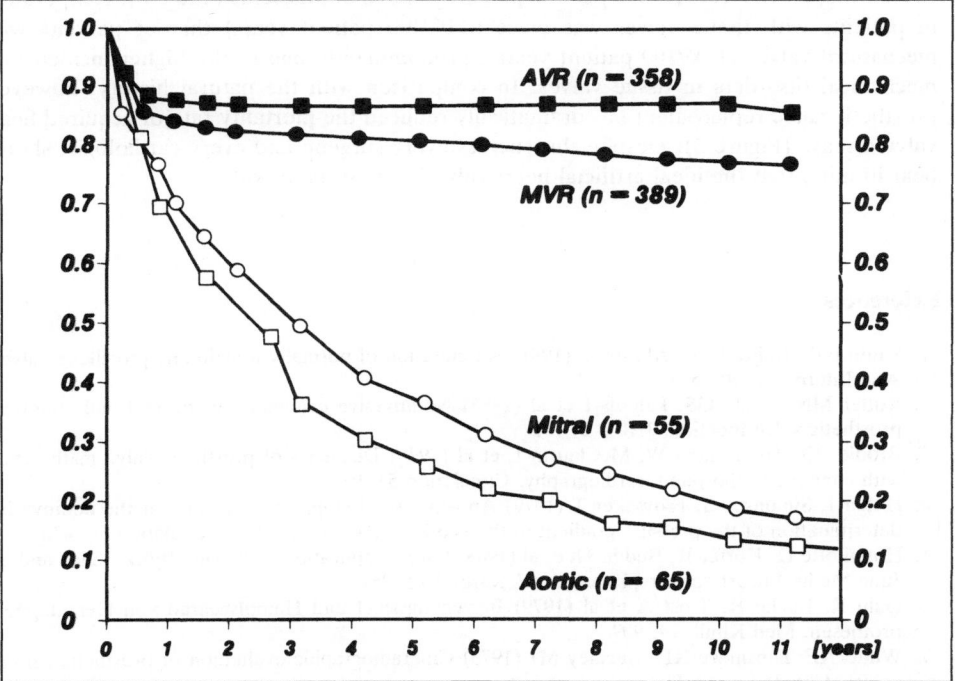

Fig. 3. Cumulative survival rates in medically and operatively treated patients with severe aortic or mitral valve lesions. AVR = aortic valve replacement group; MVR = mitral valve replacement group; Mitral = medically treated patients with mitral valve lesions NYHA III or IV; Aortic = medically treated patients with severe aortic valve lesions. The recommended operation was not performed in the conservatively treated patients for various reasons (lack of operative capacity, refusal by the patient or the surgeon).

emergency in cases with a more acute onset of symptoms. A sudden prosthetic breakdown requires immediate diagnosis with urgent surgical treatment.

Tissue ingrowth

Excessive endothelial ingrowth can interfere with valve action. The clinical features are similar to those of valvular thrombosis. A stenotic murmur, due to ingrowth into the orifice ring, is heard in more than 80% of the patients (Table 3). With the new inert materials which are of acceptable tissue compatibility, the incidence of this complication has dropped markedly. In our series we have only seen four cases during the last 10 years. Tissue ingrowth is a rather unusual preoperative diagnosis and is usually confirmed after histological examination of the explanted valve. Patients with this type of malfunction deteriorate slowly and in general, there is no need for emergency reoperation. The results of reoperation are comparable to those with uncomplicated valvular thrombosis.

Incidence of prosthetic valve malfunction

Despite all the efforts and ideas of engineers, physicians and manufacturers, complications after heart valve replacement remain a substantial source of morbidity and mortality. The overall reoperation rate is 1.12 per 100 patient years in our patients (Table 6). Reoperation in patients with tissue valves was twice (2.02/100 patient years) that of patients with mechanical valves (1.06/100 patient years), predominantly due to the higher incidence of mechanical disorders in tissue valves. In comparison with the natural history, however, prosthetic valve replacement has dramatically reduced the mortality rate of acquired heart valve disease (Figure 3). Despite this success every surgeon and every cardiologist should bear in mind that the ideal artificial heart valve is still to be found.

References

1. Smith ND, Raijzada V, Abrams J (1981) Auscultation of normally functioning prosthetic valves. Ann Intern Med 95: 594
2. Kotler MN, Mintz GS, Panidis I et al (1983) Noninvasive evaluation of normal and abnormal prosthetic valve function. JACC 2: 151
3. Brodie BR, Grossmann W, McClaurin L et al (1976) Diagnosis of prosthetic valve malfunction with combined echo-phonocardiography. Circulation 53: 93
4. Holen J, Simonsen S, Fröysaker T (1979) An ultrasound Doppler technique for the noninvasive determination of the pressure gradient in the Björk-Shiley mitral valve. Circulation 59: 436
5. Horstkotte D, Körfer R, Budde Th et al (1983) Late complications following Björk-Shiley and St. Jude Medical heart valve replacement. Z Kardiol 72: 251
6. Gahl K. Lücke R, Trost A et al (1979) Bewegungsspiel und Hämolysegrad von Herzklappen-prothesen. Med Klinik 74: 909
7. White AF, Dinsmore RE, Buckley MJ (1973) Cineradiographic evaluation of prosthetic cardiac valves. Circulation 48: 882
8. Sands MK, Lachman AS, O'Reilly et al (1982) Diagnostic value of cinefluoroscopy in the evaluation of prosthetic heart valve dysfunction. Am Heart J 104: 622
9. Kotler MN, Segae BL, Parry WR (1978) Echocardiographic and phonocardiographic evaluation of prosthetic heart valves. Cardiovasc Clin 9: 187
10. Mintz GS, Kotler MN, Steiner RM et al (1981) Ultrasonography of prosthetic cardiac valves. Crit Rev Diagn Imag 14: 243

11. Horstkotte D, Aul C, Seipel L et al (1983) Influence of valve type and valve function on chronic intravascular hemolysis following mitral and aortic valve replacement using alloprostheses. Z Kardiol 72: 119
12. Horstkotte D, Haerten K, Leuner Chr et al (1978) Chronic intravascular hemolysis following mitral valve replacement with Björk-Shiley, Lillehei-Kaster and Starr-Edwards prostheses. Z Kardiol 67: 629
13. Bokrow JC, LaGrange LD, Schoen FJ (1973) Control of structure of carbon for use in bioingeneering, chemistry, and physics of carbon. In: Walker PL (ed) Chemistry and Biophysics of Carbon, Vol 9. Marcel Dekker, New York, p 103
14. Forfar JC (1979) A 7-year analysis of hemorrhage in patients on long-term anticoagulant treatment. Br Heart J 42: 128
15. Quenzer RW, Edwards ED, Levine S (1976) A comparative study of 48 heart valve and 24 prosthetic valve endocarditis cases. Am Heart J 92: 15
16. Slaughter L, Morris JE, Starr A (1973) Prosthetic valvular endocarditis. A 12-year review. Circulation 47: 1319
17. Masur H., Johnson WD (1980) Prosthetic valve endocarditis. J Thorac Cardiovasc Surg 80: 31
18. Horstkotte D, Körfer R, Loogen F et al (1984) Prosthetic valve endocarditis: Clinical findings and management. Eur Heart J 5 (Suppl C) 117
19. Horstkotte D, Körfer R (1983) Prosthetic valve endocarditis with embolization of a Smeloff-Cutter aortic valve prosthesis: Diagnosis, operative management, and clinical and hemodynamic findings up to 3 years postoperatively. Z Kardiol 72: 476
20. Saffle JR, Gardner P, Schoenbaum SC et al (1977) Prosthetic valve endocarditis. The case for prompt replacement. J Thorac Cardiovasc Surg 73: 416
21. Brubakk O, Simonsen S, Källman L et al (1981) Strut fracture in the new Björk-Shiley mitral valve prosthesis. Thorac Cardiovasc Surg 29: 108
22. Hylen JC, Koster FE, Starr A et al (1970) Aortic ball variance: Diagnosis and treatment. Ann Int Med 72: 1
23. Joyce LD, Emery RW, Nicoloff DM (1978) Ball variance and fracture of mitral valve prosthesis causing recurrent thrombemboli. J Thorac Cardiovasc Surg 75: 309
24. Zombro GL, Cundey PE, Fishback ME et al (1977) Strut fracture in DeBakey valve. Successful reoperation and valve replacement. J Thorac Cardiovasc Surg 74: 469
25. McEnany MT, Wheeler EO, Austin WG (1979) Survival following fracture of strut from mitral prosthesis with translocation. J Thorac Cardiovasc Surg 78: 136
26. Silver MD (1980) Wear in Björk-Shiley heart valve prostheses recovered at necropsy or operation. J Thorac Cardiovasc Surg 79: 693
27. Elliott RA (1976) Björk-Shiley prosthesis recall. Circulation 53: 206
28. Fishbein MC, Gissen SA, Collins JJ et al (1977) Pathologic findings after cardiac valve replacement with glutaraldehyde-fixed porcine valves. Am J Cardiol 40: 331
29. Schoen FJ, Collins JJ, Cohn LH (1983) Long-term failure rate and morphologic correlations in porcine bioprosthetic heart valves. Am J Cardiol 51: 957
30. Ferrans VJ, Spray TL, Billingham ME et al (1984) Structural changes in glutaraldehyde-treated porcine heterografts used as substitute cardiac valves. Transmission and scanning electron microscopic observations in 12 patients. Am J Cardiol 41: 1159

Authors' address:
Professor Reiner Körfer
Direktor der Chirurgischen
Abteilung des
Herzzentrums Nordrhein-Westfalen
Georgstraße
4970 Bad Oeynhausen
F.R.G.

Valve Replacement in Children with Congenital Heart Disease

C. L. Sainz

Cardiac valve anomalies, either isolated or associated with other cardiac lesions, are frequently encountered in a pediatric cardiology practice. In each case, presenting clinical features are serious, and if the child needs a valve replacement, all the drawbacks of the prostheses add to each case's complexity.

It is not easy to define a homogenous group of children when establishing the parameters of a study. Definition of the age range of patients to whom we refer as children is not easy. Also, we are dealing with diverse conditions amenable to treatment with a valve replacement. Furthermore, correlation with other studies is difficult because the abundant publications on valve replacement in children show results by different age subsets, and at times, report acquired and inborn valve diseases together.

In our public health care system, the age limit for patient admittance to children's hospitals has been 7 years (with only a few exceptions) so our experience has been mainly with patients under age 7, which means that most of our patients have congenital malformations. A rheumatic valvular lesion at this early age is extremely rare.

Some important points concerning valve replacement, particularly relevant when one deals with a child, are the type of prosthesis and the most suitable protective postoperative medication.

Selection of valve prosthesis

The size and variation of the ventricular chambers through the cardiac cycle determine which type of valvular device should be used. Design and dimensions are important, for it is not unusual to find small, hypertrophic cavities. The best fitting models will be those with the least possible amount of protruding prosthetic material (fixed or mobile), a requirement that is met chiefly by the low profile mechanical prostheses as opposed to the cage-ball types. Biological valves have three struts which have to be accomodated within the ventricular cavity and which occasionally touch the ventricular walls during systolic contraction. Discs of the various mechanical valves also protrude into the ventricular lumen but because of their round shape, eccentric disc excursion, larger distance to the ventricular walls, and central maximal profile, contact with the ventricular walls is less likely. One more consideration to bear in mind is that with the mechanical prosthetic valves, contact at the annular level will take place at two lateral sites, and with the bioprostheses it will occur at three points. This circumstance increases the difficulty during orientation of the device in keeping a good distance between the struts and the ventricular walls. The tilting-disc prosthesis, in the maximal opening position, can also encroach onto some part of the ventricular wall; but for this to happen, the size of the ventricular cavity would have to be quite small. A stent-mounted bioprosthesis would undoubtedly also have the same trouble. In the aortic or pulmonary positions, structures surrounding the artificial valve are fixed and do not vary in

131

diameter during cardiac contraction. This allows good functioning of a cage-ball valve or a valve with long struts.

Durability and disadvantages pertaining to valve materials are in our opinion crucial elements in making the best choice. The important matter of securing good valve performance without restrictions can be accomplished satisfactorily, but a valve implies the introduction of foreign material into the circulatory system, and we should make sure that these devices will be durable and minimize, or not cause serious side effects in the patient.

Mechanical valves are much more durable than the majority of the biological valves; it is well-established that the rates of alteration, calcification and deterioration are high for tissue valves, which accounts for the high percentage that must be replaced within a short time, in contrast to a very low rate of mechanical failures. From our standpoint, this circumstance warrants the exclusion of biological prosthetic valves for use in children and especially, in infants.

We do not mean to say that mechanical valves do not fail, but failure is much more common with tissue valves. Mechanical devices are superior in stability and long-term durability, as well as in structural properties and design.

The thrombotic phenomenon, its production and location, is an eventuality and should always be considered in every valve replacement, regardless of the type of prosthesis.

Thrombus formation arises from an alteration of the vascular endothelium or endocardium, which elicits the accumulation of platelets and clot formation. Endothelial lesion or alteration will always follow, whatever prosthesis is in place, because of the native valve resection and placement of sutures. Consequently, both mechanical and biological valves facilitate conditions for the development of clots. Various materials utilized in their manufacture possess different thrombogenic potential that will accordingly modulate the outcome. In the biological devices, the metallic or rigid parts which are made of various materials are unexposed in contrast to mechanical valves.

For some time it was generally believed that bioprostheses have a low thrombogenicity which made anticoagulation therapy unnecessary. This was certainly a major advantage; however, a large series of patients with longer follow-up periods has revealed the high thrombogenic rate of these tissue valves and, consequently, the need for an anticoagulation treatment. This is due to the same lesions that promote the initiation and localization of thrombus formation on the atrioventricular endocardium and to the sewing cuff of synthetic material.

We cannot deny our preference for mechanical prostheses. We agree they offer an increased durability, are easier to orient, are less traumatic and entail no greater thrombogenicity. Degeneration and early calcification in infancy and childhood as well as the fragility and similar thrombogenic capability, put bioprostheses at a clear disadvantage, particularly at age 7 and under. We use low profile mechanical valves in the mitral and tricuspid positions. Though we do not reject the cage-ball types, we prefer low profile devices in the aortic position. We rarely insert any valve in the pulmonary position.

Postoperative treatment

Let us not forget the jeopardy of anticoagulation regimens, as well as the common hindrances to achieving proper control: the difficulties in dose adjustment aimed at maintaining the most *efficient* prothrombin times (as measured by the one-stage Quick method) and the long distance separating some patients from the control centers. The

Table 1. Problems related to anticoagulation in infancy

Difficulties in :	– Dose adjustment
	– Blood sampling
	– Controls
Bleeding	

Table 2. Problems related to anticoagulation in children

Haemarthrosis
Epistaxis
Other bleeding complications
Wounds

dangers of excessive anticoagulation override the risk of thromboembolism without anticoagulants. Fluctuation in dosage gives rise to great variations in prothrombin time measurements and temporary interruption of treatment causes acute thrombembolic complications. A therapeutic scheme yielding prothrombin time determinations not corresponding to those regarded as effective will be incorrect or mildly protective.

In our clinical environment, confined to the child and infant under school age, the inconvenience and risks associated with anticoagulation are quite apparent (see Tables 1 and 2). On the one hand, fragmentation of tablets will never provide the precise age-related dose and, on the other hand, both the infant and the preschool child, apart from the dangers of bleeding because of faulty or inadequate adjustment of dose, are at a high risk of sustaining traumatic hemorrhages that may occur far away from the hospital.

With this in mind, we decided to try out the antiplatelet drugs (1,2). Young patients were started on easy-to-follow antiaggregation regimens immediately after the first postoperative hours. This significantly decreased the hazards of hemorrhage and afforded prevention of thrombotic complications. Endothelial lesions, the early anatomical basis for the aggregation of platelets and the starting point for the development of thrombi, would be protected by such treatment.

Our current treatment protocol is: patients with an aortic valve prosthesis do not receive any drug therapy; patients with a mitral or tricuspid prosthesis are placed temporarily on acetyl-salicylic acid plus dipyramidole. This regimen is maintained for 6 months, which is long enough for the endothelial lesions to become completely repaired. Then the regimen is discontinued in all cases.

Indications

A valve replacement in an infant must take into consideration the position of the prosthesis and whether this valvular replacement should be performed or deferred until all other reparative or conservative methods have failed. Another consideration is whether partial repair will bring enough hemodynamic improvement to allow postponement of valve replacement until the patient's age is more suitable for a satisfactory correction. The size of the prosthesis will depend on the child's age and body surface, and to a variable extent on the type and severity of the valve lesion. Insertion of as large a size as possible will minimize the need for reoperation as the child grows. Unfortunately, this cannot always be

Table 3. Valve replacement

Surgical indications
– Heart failure not compensated with medical treatment – Postoperative heart failure – Syncopes due to aortic valve stenosis – Progressive cardiac enlargement – Episodes of acute pulmonary edema

accomplished but we replace a valve whenever we are certain that this approach represents the best alternative for the child's recovery.

It is undoubtedly hard to establish therapeutic patterns for pediatric cases of valve anomalies, since isolated lesions in the child are less common and usually occur as part of many complex conditions. The derangement and hemodynamic embarrassment will depend upon multiple factors (see Table 3). We include as candidates for valve replacement patients who follow a downhill course despite medical management, with persistent congestive failure, syncopes, acute episodes of pulmonary edema, progressive cardiac enlargement and greatly deteriorated general physical conditions. This surgical approach may be extended to those cases of truncus arteriosus communis with truncal valve incompetence and the acute iatrogenic insufficiencies of the mitral and aortic valves.

Patients in the study

Between February 1974 and September 1983, 36 patients underwent a valve replacement operation; in all cases a Björk-Shiley® prosthesis was inserted in all three – mitral, aortic, or tricuspid – positions. We have not used any other type of artificial valve. There were 8 AVR, 26 MVR, and 2 TVR. The ages of patients ranged from 4 months to 8 years, with 8 cases under one year; operative mortality reached 11.1% (4 patients) (see Table 4).

Results

We realize that our case series, because of its low number of patients and short follow-up time, does not permit valid or definitive conclusions; and the great variety of diagnoses and clinical procedures make it difficult to separate patients into homogeneous groups.

However, we believe that it can point to the experience a larger number of children with a valve prosthesis will undergo. Our actuarial survival curve (see Figure 1) shows a large standard error of ± 28% with a 9-year survival of 58.2%, which is not indicative.

Table 4. Valve replacement Feb. 74 – Sep. 83

Björk-Shiley valves			
4 months	– 12 months	8	(1)
1 yr	– 3 yrs	9	(1)
3 yrs	– 6 yrs	12	(1)
6 yrs	– 8 yrs	7	(1)
		36 (4)	11.1%

( ) deaths

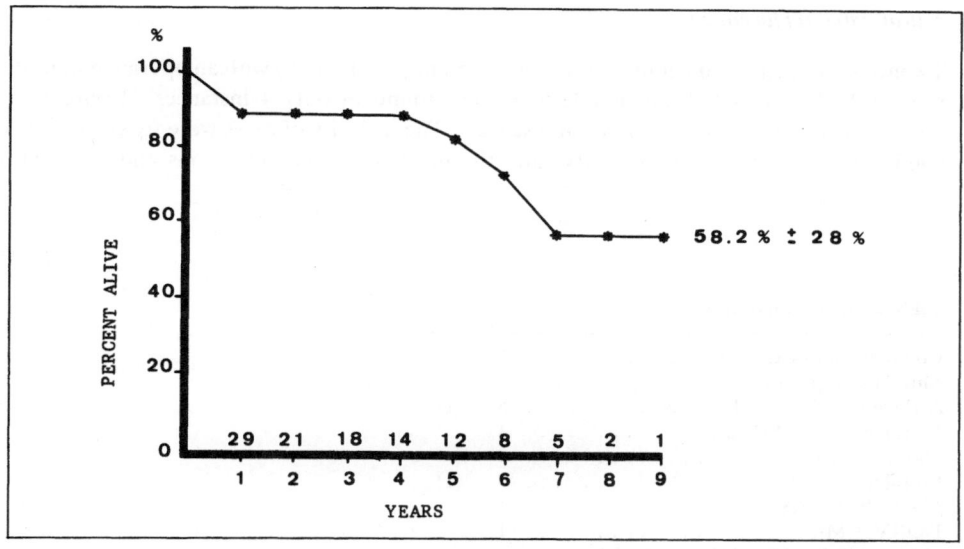

Fig. 1. Actuarial survival curve of children with a valve prosthesis

Aortic valve replacement

Aortic incompetence occurs infrequently in pediatric years, and therefore requires few valve prostheses. In our experience (see Table 5) with 8 patients there were no deaths or complications (including thromboembolism).

A patient with a 17 mm aortic prosthesis inserted in 1975 (at 4 years of age) is now waiting for a larger prosthesis because he has developed aortic stenosis.

The larger sizes (27 mm and 29 mm) are mitral, and inserted from the ventricular side at the time of correction of truncus arteriosus. None of these children whose ages ranged between 4 and 8 years has received anticoagulation or antiplatelet therapies.

The ages of the patients on whom we performed an aortic valve replacement were older than patients who underwent a mitral replacement.

Table 5. Aortic valve replacement

	Number	Size
Combined aortic disease	2	19–19
Aortic incompetence	1	17
Truncus arteriosus type I	1	27 M
Truncus arteriosus type II	1	29 M
Tetralogy of Fallot + AI	1	19
Aortic stenosis (Konno)	1	21
Iatrogenic (CASD)	1	17
	8	

AI=Aortic insufficiency. CASD=Complete atrio-ventricular septal defects. M=Mitral.

Mitral valve replacement

Twenty-six patients had a mitral valve replacement (see Table 6) with an operative mortality rate of 11.1%. Isolated valvular lesions were found in only 4 instances (2 pure mitral insufficiencies and 2 combined mitral diseases). The majority of cases were from a variety of conditions. Despite a low mortality rate, the incidence of complications and reoperation

Table 6. Mitral valve replacements

Combined mitral disease	2	
Mitral incompetence	2	
Atrioventricular septal defects	5	(1)
Mitral lesion + VSD	4	
Shone syndrome	3	
Mitral lesion + EF	3	(1)
MS + VSD + AS	1	
DORV + MI.	1	
TGA + VSD + PS + MI (iatrogenic)	1	
Mitral lesion + HSS	1	(1)
Senning procedure + MI	1	
Corrected transposition + TI	1	
Corrected transposition + VSD + TI	1	
	26	(3)

VSD=ventricular septal defect. EF=endocardial fibroelastosis. MS=mitral stenosis. AS=aortic stenosis. DORV-=double outlet right ventricle. MI=mitral insufficiency. TGA=transposition of the great arteries. PS=pulmonary stenosis. HSS=hypertrophic subaortic stenosis. TI=tricuspid insufficiency. Figures in parentheses are deaths.

Table 7. Reoperations on the mitral valve.

No. of patients. 23		
No. reoperations 10	43.4%	
	12.1 ± 3.8% patient-year	
Causes of reoperation:		
Perivalvular aneurysm.		2
Dehiscence.		1
Pacemaker		1
Causes of re-replacement:	Valve no.	
Syndrome of mitral stenosis 1	19–23	
Panus 2	3–25 cleaning	
Thrombosis 2	21–25 29–29	
Fibrothrombosis 1	17–19	

136

Table 8. Tricuspid valve replacement

Mustard procedure + TI .	1	
Ebstein	1	(1)
	2	(1)

TI=Tricuspid insufficiency.
Figure in parentheses is death.

Table 9. Early and late mortality after valve replacement

Parameters	No.	% death (linear)	% death per pat.-yr. $\bar{x}$	SEM
Hospital deaths	4	11.1	–	–
Late deaths causes:	6	18.7	7.3	± 2.9
Fibroelastosis	2	6.2	2.4	± 1.7
Reoperation	2	6.2	2.4	± 1.7
Valvular obstruction by panus	1	3.1	1.2	± 1.2
Unknown	1	3.1	1.2	± 1.2

rates have been high, up to 43.2% (12.1 ± 3.8%) per patient year (see Table 7), because of the severity and complexity of the patients' preoperative conditions.

Thromboembolic complications

No early thrombosis was recorded in this group of patients who were put on antiaggregation regimens over a 6-month period. Late thrombotic events occurred at 18 and 72 months representing 3.6 ± 2.1% per patient year. Reoperations were needed to replace the malfunctioning prostheses because of thrombosis in 3 cases and pannus overgrowth in 2 cases. On another occasion, the size of the initial prosthesis had already become too small for the patient's body surface. With the exception of the patient who had a 29 mm prosthesis replaced with a new one of the same size, in the remainder we were able to insert a prosthetic valve one or two sizes larger.

When to replace an artificial valve in children remains a question of the valve's relatively small size, and this issue will need further experience.

Tricuspid valve replacement

Only 2 patients received a tricuspid valve prosthesis (see Table 8).

Late mortality

In only one case did the cause of death remain unknown; the others are listed in Table 9.

References

1. Weinstein GS, Mavroudis C, Ebert PA (1982) Preliminary experience with aspirin for anticoagulation in children with prosthetic cardiac valves. Ann Thorac Surg 33:549
2. Pass HI, Sade RM, Crawford FA et al (1984) Cardiac valve prostheses in children without anticoagulation. J Thorac Cardiovasc Surg 87:832

Author's address:

C. L. Sainz, M. D.
Servico de Ciruvogia
Residencia Sanitaria Valle d'Hebron
Barcelona
Spain

Valve Replacement in Infancy and Childhood

T. E. Kersten, D. M. Nicoloff, K. V. Arom,
W. G. Lindsay and W. F. Northrup

The basic philosophy of valve replacement in the pediatric age group has not changed over the past years: preservation of autologous tissue valves within the confines/constraints of appropriate retained hemodynamic function of the native valve. Although several valve models and types have surfaced in the past five years, it has now become clear and generally accepted that tissue heart valves are currently inappropriate in the pediatric age group. This limitation of the biologic valve in the younger age group stems primarily from the lack of durability and hence longevity of the valve, irrespective of its anatomical position.

There is obviously no perfect valve. However, on the basis of
1. low geometric profile,
2. low thrombogenicity,
3. currently unsurpassed hemodynamics with central laminar flow, particularly in the smaller prosthetic valve diameter sizes (< 23 mm) and
4. proven durability,
   we have chosen the St. Jude Medical (SJM) prosthesis as the valve of choice in the pediatric age group.

Surgical experience with the St. Jude Medical valve in the pediatric age group

This report relates our own experience with valve replacement in children with the St. Jude valve from 1978 to 1984.

Fifteen patients underwent valve replacement with a mean age of 10.7 years. Four patients were less than 2.5 years old. In our small group, 60% (n=9) of the patients had a diagnosis of valvular disease only whereas 40% (n=6) had complex problems. Of the three patients who eventually required a mitral valve replacement (MVR) secondary to an earlier procedure, two of these were complete A–V canals with subsequently severe mitral insufficiency after the primary repair. Table 1 shows the distribution of the patients as well as the associated hospital mortality with an overall mortality of 13%.

One death was in a 17-month-old infant who had been referred in extremis after aortic valvotomy for congenital aortic stenosis with severe aortic insufficiency and angiographic findings of severe endocardial fibroelastosis. A Konno-Rastan procedure (1) was performed to allow placement of a 19 mm SJM aortic prosthesis. The second death was in a 2-year-old infant with severe mitral regurgitation after complete repair of an AV-canal defect. The child was in severe biventricular failure and required a 19 mm St. Jude Medial mitral prosthesis, which was inserted via a transatrial septal approach. The infant died in the immediate postoperative period from multiorgan failure. Autopsy demonstrated the valve in an appropriate position with normal function.

Table 1. Pediatric operative mortality

	No. of cases	No. of deaths	%
AVR	5	0	0
AVR + Misc.	2	1	50
MVR	4	1	25
MVR + Misc.	3	0	0
DVR (AVR + MVR)	1	0	0
Total	15	2	13

The average valve size used was 27 mm in the mitral position with the exception of a 27-month-old and a 6-month-old patient in whom 19 mm prostheses were used. Similarly with the aortic position, the average valve size was 25 mm except in two patients of 17 months and 6 months in whom 19 mm prostheses were placed.

The patient requiring double valve (AVR + MVR) replacement deserves special comment. A 6-months-old 5.6 kg female was referred in extremis after aortic valvotomy for congenital aortic stenosis. The patient developed massive aortic regurgitation and also had severe mitral regurgitation secondary to an infarcted papillary muscle seen at the time of valve replacement. The infant underwent AVR and MVR with two 19 mm SJM aortic prostheses. The aortic prosthesis was chosen for the mitral position because of the small sewing skirt and limited confines of the left atrium. The mitral anulus and aortic ring were enlarged posteriorly with the Manouguian procedure (2, 3); the aortic ring was opened anteriorly with the Konno-Rastan operation to accomodate the 19 mm valve since the aortic ring was hypoplastic. Bovine pericardium was used to reconstruct the roof of the left atrium, interventricular septum, the right ventricular outflow tract and the ascending aorta (4).

Our surgical technique employs systemic hypothermia with crystalloid potassium cardio-plegic arrest as indicated, as well as topical hypothermia when possible. In the infants, we seat the valves with a running suture technique with a monofilament polypropylene suture, whereas in the older age group we traditionally use interrupted mattress sutures placed around the sewing ring. Core temperature is lowered to 25–28 °C.

Anticoagulation in infants and children with prosthetic valves

The subject of anticoagulation in the pediatric age group with prosthetic heart valves is currently under investigation. Our personal choice is to anticoagulate all patients having prosthetic valves in the aortic or mitral position with a warfarin derivative, even in the pediatric age group. Although some people claim that the use of warfarin imposes undue

Table 2. Number of emboli

AVR	0
AVR + Misc.	1
MVR	0
MVR + Misc.	0
DVR + Misc.	0

Incidence of thrombembolic events = 2.7/100 pt. yrs.

hardship and strain on the parents, infant and pediatrician, we have not found this to be prohibitive to its use. Prothrombin times (protimes) are kept at about 1.5–2 times the control level for valves in the aortic and mitral positions. The use of warfarin has resulted in only one documented case of thromboembolism in an 18-year-old patient with a SJM valve in the aortic position and an ascending aortic graft placed for acute dissection. The overall thromboembolic incidence was 2.7/100 patient-years in our pediatric group (see Table 2). This one patient with the embolus had a normal protime at the time of the event.

Weinstein et al (5) have treated twelve pediatric patients having mechanical prostheses with aspirin plus dipyridamole and concluded that this drug regimen provided adequate and acceptable protection against thromboembolism and avoided the hemorrhagic complications associated with warfarin. We had initially adopted this tactic in the 6-month-old patient with the AVR + MVR in the hope of avoiding the blood work for protimes. The infant returned 2 months postoperatively in consecutive heart failure secondary to a partially thrombosed mitral valve. An intravenous urokinase infusion was started at 4000 units/kg/h for 18 hours with resolution of the congestive heart failure and return of the mitral valve function to normal as documented by fluoroscopy. The infant was subsequently switched to warfarin therapy with continued normal development at 18 months postoperatively. The substantial amount of bovine pericardium used in the reconstruction of the heart may have added significantly to the thrombogenic millieu and resulted in the thrombus formation.

A recent report by Pass, Sade, et al. (6) involves 34 children in whom the St. Jude valve is being followed without any form of antiocoagulation. These investigators claim that, to date, the results are as good as or better than their previous experience with warfarin in regard to thromboembolic complications. The two exceptions by these investigators are: presence of atrial fibrillation or use of the SJM valve in the tricuspid position. The issue which valve should be used in the tricuspid position, i.e., St. Jude Medical or tissue valves, is far from settled. In any event, this report gives credence to the very low thrombogenicity of the SJM valve, particularly in children where several factors may play a role in the low incidence of thromboembolism:

(1) Increased heart rate with rapid bileaflet motion and decreased stasis around the valve structure.
(2) Small chamber sizes in the infant heart with rapid blood flow and hence relatively less stasis.
(3) Normal sinus rhythm in a heart with a relatively small left atrial size.

We will continue to anticoagulate all our patients with warfarin until the answer becomes clear as to the best protection against thromboembolism in the pediatric age group. Also, clearly the valve of choice in infants and children is the St. Jude Medical prosthesis with its central flow, minimal gradient even in the smaller sizes, and extremely low thrombogenicity in light of proven durability. In addition, the excellent hemodynamics relative to any size of this valve should allow the child to keep the prosthetic valve for a longer time before reoperation becomes necessary.

References

1. Konno S, Imai Y, Iida Y et al (1975) A new method for prosthetic valve replacement in congenital aortic stenosis associated with hypoplasia of the aortic valve ring. J Thorac Cardiovasc Surg 70:909
2. Manouguian S, Abu-Aiskah N, Neitzel J (1979) Patch enlargement of the aortic and mitral valve rings with aortic and mitral double valve replacement. J Thorac Cardiovasc Surg 78:394

3. Rastan H, Atai M, Audi H et al (1981) Enlargement of mitral valvular ring. J Thorac Cardiovasc Surg 81:106
4. Kersten TE, Bessinger FB, Stone FM et al (1984) Combined techniques for double valve replacement in the infant. Ann Thorac Surg (in press)
5. Weinstein GS, Mavroudis C, Ebert PA (1982) Preliminary experience with aspirin for anticoagulation in children with prosthetic cardiac valves. Ann Thorac Surg 33:549
6. Pass HI, Sade RM, Crawford FA et al (1984) Cardiac valve prostheses in children without anticoagulation. J Thorac Cardiovasc Surg 87:832

Authors' address:
Thomas E. Kersten, M.D.
Minneapolis Heart Institute, Minneapolis
United Hospitals, St. Paul
Minnesota, U.S.A.

Controversies in Heart Valve Replacement

D. HORSTKOTTE, Düsseldorf · H. P. KRAYENBÜHL,
Zürich · F. LOOGEN, Düsseldorf (eds.)

1986. 360 pages. Cloth DM 120,–; US $ 45.00
ISBN 3-7985-0680-9 (Steinkopff)
ISBN 0-387-91269-X (Springer-Verlag New York)

Contents: Operative Treatment and Choice of Valve – Treatment after Heart Valve Surgery – Indication and Contraindication for Surgical Intervention – Operative Treatment and Choice of Valve – Diagnosis and Prognosis of Valvular Heart Disease – Indication and Contraindication for Surgical Intervention.

The implantation of prosthetic heart valves has a 25-year history. With this background experts in heart valve replacement gathered in Düsseldorf in May 1985 for an exchange of views, the results of which are presented in this volume. Opinions may be found on the diagnosis and prognosis of valvular lesions, indications and contraindications for surgical intervention, the choice of prosthesis, and operative and postoperative treatment.

This book is the first of its type to bring together all the essential problems of prosthesis heart valve replacement, which is still subject to controversy. The brief space of time between symposium and publication guarantees the topicality of this book.

Distribution in US and Canada through Springer-Verlag, 175 Fifth Avenue, New York, NY 10010; for other countries through your bookseller or directly from Dr. Dietrich Steinkopff Verlag, P. O. Box 11 1008, 6100 Darmstadt/West Germany.

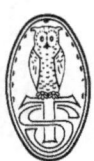 **Steinkopff Verlag Darmstadt**
Springer-Verlag New York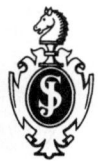

CSI – A New Approach to Interventional Cardiology

Edited by W. MOHL, Vienna / D. FAXON, Boston /
E. WOLNER, Vienna

1986. 100 pages with numerous figures and tables.
Cloth DM 48,–; US $ 19.20
ISBN 3-7985-0694-9 (Steinkopff)
ISBN 0-387-91273-8 (Springer-Verlag New York)

Contents: Report of the international working group on coronary sinus interventions – The so-called "silent zone" of the coronary sinus – Inflow, outflow and pressures in the coronary circulation – Coronary sinus interventions: Clinical application – The promise and limitation of coronary venous retroperfusion: Lessons from the past and new directions – Synchronized coronary sinus retroperfusion current clinical perspective – PICSO status report 1985 – Retrograde cardioplegia: Myocardial protection via the coronary veins – 1986 – Technical aspects of coronary sinus interventions – Pros and cons-coronary sinus intervention vs. conventional therapy – CSI: Temporary support or long-term therapy.

CSI – A New Approach to Interventional Cardiology focuses on the clinical evaluation of systems such as synchronized retroperfusion (SRP), retroinfusion of pharmaceutical agents (RCSP) and pressure controlled intermittent coronary sinus occlusion (PICSO). This first volume of the series *Progress in Coronary Sinus Interventions,* with the latest contributions on the mechanisms, pathophysiology and anatomy of the coronary venous system, together with experimental results on coronary sinus intervention, thus provides the groundwork for further discussion, research and development in this field.

Distribution in US and Canada through Springer-Verlag, 175 Fifth Avenue, New York, NY 10010; for other countries through your bookseller or directly from Dr. Dietrich Steinkopff Verlag, P. O. Box 11 1008, 6100 Darmstadt/West Germany.

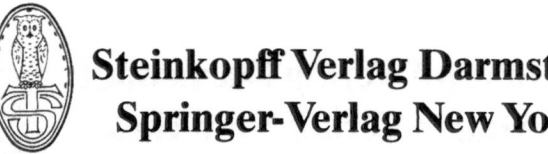 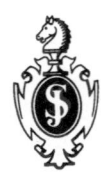

Steinkopff Verlag Darmstadt
Springer-Verlag New York

The Coronary Sinus

Proceedings of the 1st International Symposium on Myocardial Protection Via the Coronary Sinus Vienna, February 27-29, 1984

W. MOHL / E. WOLNER / D. GLOGAR (eds.)

1984. 560 pages, extensively illustrated with figures and tables.
Cloth DM 140,–; US $ 63.00
ISBN 3-7985-0634-4 (Steinkopff)
ISBN 0-387-91250-9 (Springer-Verlag New York)

Contents: 1. Anatomy and Pathophysiology of Venous System.
2. Interventions Using the Coronary Sinus Route: Intraoperative Protection Via the Coronary Sinus — Basic Physiology on Retroperfusion and Coronary Sinus Occlusion — Intermittent Coronary Sinus Occlusion Modalities — Synchronized Retroperfusion Modalities.

This book is the first to deal with the coronary sinus as an alternative access route, as part of the heart-vein system, to the diseased heart muscle.

Not only are the scientific fundamentals from biophysics, biochemistry, computer science and anatomy discussed, the latest perspectives in coronary venous anatomy and physiology, as well as technical aspects of measurements and pump systems are also dealt with. The principal aim of the book is to describe the types of interventions currently being developed which have been proved valid to protect ischemic myocardium. The papers give an account of the results from the latest experimental and clinical research. The book also focuses on techniques such as retrograde coronary sinus perfusion and coronary sinus occlusion. Of special importance are the papers on intermittent occlusion and synchronized retroperfusion modalities.

These proceedings address basic scientists in microcirculation, cardiologists, cardiac surgeons, pathologists, physiologists, anatomists, and students, for whom retroperfusion techniques via the coronary sinus may have great clinical potential.

Distribution in US and Canada through Springer-Verlag, 175 Fifth Avenue, New York, NY 10010; for other countries through your bookseller or directly from Dr. Dietrich Steinkopff Verlag, P. O. Box 11 1008, 6100 Darmstadt/West Germany.

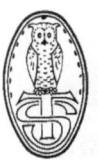 **Steinkopff Verlag Darmstadt**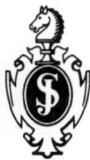
Springer-Verlag New York

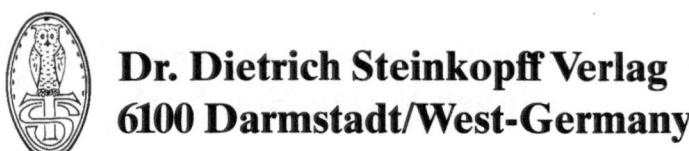